HEALTHY
AGING

ANNALS OF TRADITIONAL CHINESE MEDICINE

Series Editors: Ping-Chung Leung
(The Chinese University of Hong Kong, Hong Kong)
Charlie Changli Xue
(RMIT University, Australia)

Published

Volume 1 Chinese Medicine — Modern Practice
Edited by Ping-Chung Leung & Charlie Changli Xue
ISBN: 978-981-256-018-6
Publication date: February 2005   252 pp.

Volume 2 Current Review of Chinese Medicine: Quality Control of Herbs and Herbal Material
Edited by Ping-Chung Leung, Harry Fong & Charlie Changli Xue
ISBN: 978-981-256-707-9
Publication date: May 2006   308 pp.

Volume 3 Alternative Treatment for Cancer
Edited by Ping-Chung Leung & Harry Fong
ISBN: 978-981-270-929-5
Publication date: November 2007   384 pp.

Forthcoming

Volume 5 Evidence-Based Acupuncture
Edited by Ping-Chung Leung
ISBN: 978-981-4324-17-5
Scheduled publication date: Fall 2011   Approx. 200 pp.

HEALTHY AGING

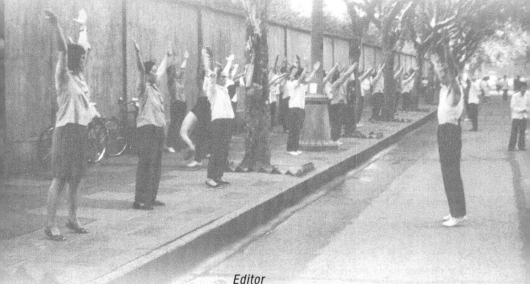

Editor

Ping-Chung Leung

The Chinese University of Hong Kong

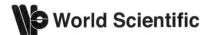

World Scientific

NEW JERSEY · LONDON · SINGAPORE · BEIJING · SHANGHAI · HONG KONG · TAIPEI · CHENNAI

Published by

World Scientific Publishing Co. Pte. Ltd.

5 Toh Tuck Link, Singapore 596224

USA office: 27 Warren Street, Suite 401-402, Hackensack, NJ 07601

UK office: 57 Shelton Street, Covent Garden, London WC2H 9HE

British Library Cataloguing-in-Publication Data
A catalogue record for this book is available from the British Library.

ISBN-13 978-981-4317-71-9
ISBN-10 981-4317-71-3

Typeset by Stallion Press
Email: enquiries@stallionpress.com

Printed in Singapore.

Contents

Contributors

Sim-Kim Cheng
Chung Hwa Medical Institution
Singapore College of Traditional Chinese Medicine
Singapore 319522

Harry H.S. Fong
Department of Medicinal Chemistry and Pharmacognosy
University of Illinois at Chicago
Chicago, IL 60612, USA

Lei Hong
School of Traditional Chinese Medicine
Chongqing Medical University
Chongqing, China

Siu-Ping Lam
Department of Psychiatry
Shatin Hospital
Shatin, New Territories, Hong Kong

Ping-Chung Leung
The Institute of Chinese Medicine
The Chinese University of Hong Kong
Shatin, New Territories, Hong Kong

Jian-Sheng Li
Gerontology Institute
Henan Traditional Chinese Medical College
Zhengzhou, Henan 450008, China

Su-Yun Li
Institute of Respiratory Disease
First Affiliated Hospital of Henan Traditional Chinese Medical College
Zhengzhou, Henan 450008, China

Song-Ming Liang
School of Chinese Medicine
The Chinese University of Hong Kong
Shatin, New Territories, Hong Kong

Zhi-Xiu Lin
School of Chinese Medicine
The Chinese University of Hong Kong
Shatin, New Territories, Hong Kong

Lin-Lin Liu
Key Lab for Supramolecular Structure and Materials
Jilin University, Changchun 130012, China

Gail Mahady
Department of Pharmacy Practice
PAHO/WHO Collaborating Center for Traditional Medicine
College of Pharmacy, University of Illinois at Chicago
Chicago, IL 60612, USA

Rudolf Moldzio
Institute for Medical Chemistry
Veterinary Medical University
Vienna 1210, Austria

Khaled Radad
Department of Pathology, Faculty of Veterinary Medicine
Assiut University, Assiut 71526, Egypt

Wolf-Dieter Rausch
Institute for Medical Chemistry
Department of Natural Sciences
University of Veterinary Medicine Vienna
Vienna 1210, Austria

Shirley Telles
Swami Vivekananda Yoga Research Foundation
Bangalore, India

Naveen K. Visweswaraiah
Foundation for Assessment and Integration of
    Traditional Health Systems [FAITHS]
Bengaluru, India

Ming-Hang Wang
Gerontology Institute
Henan Traditional Chinese Medical College
Zhengzhou, Henan 450008, China

Yun-Kwok Wing
Department of Psychiatry
The Chinese University of Hong Kong
Shatin, New Territories, Hong Kong

Chun-Bo Xu
World Federation of Chinese Medicine Societies
Xianlin University City
Nanjing, Jiangsu Province, 210029 China

Xue-Qing Yu
Gerontology Institute
Henan Traditional Chinese Medical College
Zhengzhou, Henan 450008, China

Xiang-Yong Zhang
World Federation of Chinese Medicine Societies
Xianlin University City
Nanjing, Jiangsu Province, 210029 China

Preface to Series

Does Traditional Chinese Medicine Work?

History should be acknowledged and respected. Despite this, the historical value of Chinese medicine in China and some parts of Asia should not be used as the only important evidence of efficacy.

While clinical science has followed closely the principles of deductive research in science and developed its methodology of wide acceptance, there is a natural demand from both users and service providers that the same methodology be applied to the traditional art of healing. There should be only one scale for the measurement of efficacy. Thus, evidence-based medicine, which apparently is the only acceptable form of treatment, would also claim its sovereignty in Chinese medicine.

In spite of influential proponents and diligent practitioners, efforts relating to the application of evidence-based medicine methodology to Chinese medicine research have been slow and unimpressive. This should not come as a surprise. Evidence-based medicine requires the knowledge of the exact chemistry of the drug used, the exact physical or chemical activities involved and above all, the biological responses in the recipient. All these are not known. Working back from the black box of old historical records of efficacy requires huge resources and time, if at all possible. Insistence on this approach would result in either unending frustrations or utter desperation.

Parallel with the modern attempts, respectable Chinese medicine practitioners have unendingly and relentlessly cried out their objection to the evidence-based approach. They insisted that all the evidences were already there from the Classical Records. Forcing the classical applications through a rigid modern framework of scrutiny is artificially coating Chinese medicine with a scientific clothing that does not fit.

Thus, the modern proponents are facing an impasse when they rely totally on modern scientific concepts. The traditional converts are persisting to push their pilgrims of defense. Where do we stand so as to achieve the best results of harmonisation?

There must be a compromise somewhere. Classic evidences can be transformed into a universal language to be fairly evaluated and to be decided whether suitable for further research, using the deductive methodology or an innovative one after intelligent modifications.

There is a need for a platform on which a direction can be developed in the attempt to modernise the traditional art and science of healing, while remaining free and objective to utilise the decaying wisdom without prejudice.

With the growing demand for complementary/alternative medicine from the global public and a parallel interest from the service providers, there is an urgent need for the provision of valuable information in this area.

The Annals of Chinese Medicine is a timely serial publication responding to this need. It will be providing authoritative and current information about Chinese medicine in the areas of clinical trials, biological activities of herbs, education, research and quality control requirements. Contributors are invited to send in their reports and reviews to ensure quality and value. Clinicians and scientists who are willing to submit their valuable observations, resulting from their painstaking researches are welcome to send in their manuscripts. *The Annals of Chinese Medicine* has the objective of providing a lasting platform for all who concentrate their efforts on the modernization of Chinese medicine.

Professor Ping-Chung Leung
Institute of Chinese Medicine
The Chinese University of Hong Kong

Preface to Volume 4

The fourth volume of the *Annals of Traditional Chinese Medicine* is dedicated to Aging. With affluency the projected lifespan of people in every developed or developing country increases. Longevity is considered a blessing worldwide, more emphatically among the Oriental communities. Living a long and healthy life is on everyone's wish list, whereas being an elderly with chronic diseases and multiple degenerative areas is our greatest fear. From the socio-economic perspective, caring for an ever-growing elderly population is in itself a highly challenging responsibility on both community and government levels. Caring for the same number of unhealthy individuals will be an almost impossible task.

Ever since the elderly boom has become real, health providers and bioscientists have been directing a lot of resources to the maintenance of health for the elderlies. Aging and degeneration are coupled facts. Deterioration of physical ability leads to frailty. If there are ways to slow down degeneration and practices to maintain physical ability, general and widespread promotion should start immediately.

Oriental societies have a long history of promoting health by preventing disease, which are not short of special terms and connotations. Thus for traditional Chinese medicine (TCM), "treating diseases before its onset" does not refer to what we understand by the Public Health Standard of disease prevention, but points to a more personalized pursuit of good health before the individual is disease-stricken. Under this category of medical practice, living and eating habits, lifestyles and special supplements, are all included. In fact TCM practitioners consider food to be a form of medicine. The Indians are equally conscious about lifestyle and diet.

The Oriental concept of health is gradually being recognized by the affluent societies in the US and Europe to different degrees as are apparent from the rising popularities of Oriental health supplements and exercises. However, with the highly developed advances in science, the main approach to geriatrics is still geared towards scientific discoveries and technological interventions which are linked with new enterprises.

Different commercial health promotion groups and societies have emerged in the past ten to 15 years, offering high-level investigations for people who are elderly or have reached a certain age, to "rule-out" causes of ailment. Logically speaking, ailments may not be felt (symptomatic), but probably will further deteriorate into illnesses. These health enterprises label the ailments as mild or subclinical deficiencies, or excesses. The manifestations can be related to exocrine glands, hence causing gastrointestinal ailments; or working through endocrine systems, thus producing minor hormonal disturbances. Likewise food allergy is equated with toxicity, or subclinical toxicities which are assumed to be affecting the whole individual, not only confined to the digestive system. Sophisticated laboratory tests are required because the clinical laboratories are capable of detecting only gross deficiencies, excesses and toxicities. The highly specialized tests are aimed only at amino and organic acids, which are carbohydrate metabolism markers, methylation pathway markers, antioxidant markers, intestinal dysbiosis markers, fatty acid metabolism markers, etc. These highly specific chemicals are detected from the individual's blood or urine samples. These groups of clinicians and bio-scientists have extrapolated their laboratory knowledge to the clinic; so when a certain metabolic pathway goes off track, they come to expect some marker change. However, there are those of us who realize that our day-to-day physiology is actually a dynamic process that constantly changes and yet is maintained in a broad level of balance or harmony. They have doubts on whether a unique, queer, minor diversion from the normal pathway is serious enough to warrant treatment. Thus, the new health enterprises targeting towards minor metabolic changes can be charged with the engagement in medicalization.

It is therefore the intention of this book to devote the contents to the Oriental way of maintaining elderly health: from the general concepts, to eating habits; from botanical supplements, herbal medicine, to natural healing in China and India. Some specific considerations are given to some areas like neurodegeneration, sleep disorders, pulmonary obstruction and dental problems. Perhaps the best way to prepare for a healthy longevity is to be able to formulate a do-it-yourself program.

As always the Editors are most grateful to the generous contributions of the authors.

Professor Ping-Chung Leung
Institute of Chinese Medicine
The Chinese University of Hong Kong

Chapter 1

Healthy Aging: Western and Oriental Means of Accomplishment

Ping-Chung Leung

Abstract

Modern medicine has developed along a deductive pathway which advocates the identification of the cause of a disease entity, thence create a technique to clear the pathology. Chemical drugs are often involved in this process of target-shooting, which has been very successful when a disease has a single straightforward cause.

Aging involves complicated degenerative changes which cannot be corrected by simple removal or counteractions. Aging is affecting large populations and has become a public health problem. Developing multiple methodologies counteracting aging is an important issue for health providers. A new stream of clinicians has started special aging clinics in Europe and United States to give special services to the elderly who complain about fatigue, loss of energy and general malaise. This group assumes that those aging syndromes are the result of subtle hormonal deficiencies or subclinical toxic states. Basing on the "bullet-shot" theory, specific hormonal supplements or detoxications for the problems. The efficacy of this approach has to be proven. On the other hand, Oriental medicine advocates prevention of disease and degeneration before symptoms are felt. This can be done with active but non-strenuous exercise training, careful choice of a balanced diet and psychosocial means to maintain an internal harmony. To facilitate this practice of natural healing and disease prevention, practitioners of Chinese medicine have used a variety of herbs, either as accompanying ingredients in daily cooking or as specific broths. The Oriental way of natural healing demands a fervent personal commitment and is recommended for all those being challenged with aging.

Keywords: Aging; Natural Healing; Ayurveda.

1.1 Introduction

Aging has been considered an issue of natural development and with aging, deterioration of physiological activities which initiate illnesses, is also considered unavoidable.

With the worldwide trend of increasing age, and the "elderly boom" (Buckwalter *et al.*, 2003), aging has emerged as a special problem both personally to the individual and to the health administrators alike (see Fig. 1.1). The individual worries that aging is linked with illnesses and physical suffering. The health administrators are more concerned with health economy which might not be able to handle the expanding need of the elderly population.

1.1.1 *Senior boom*

Patho-physiological changes leading to diseases could be unique and specific for the younger individuals and adequate treatment produces straight forward recovery. On the other hand, elderly people are facing a general decline of physiological functions which brings about multiple affections of different organs, making treatment and care complicated and difficult.

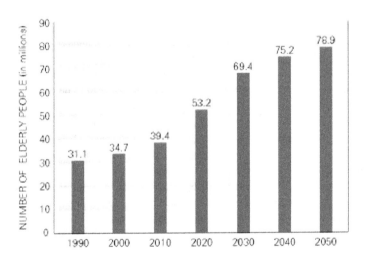

Fig. 1.1.   The Senior Boom in the US.

1.1.2 *Aging and degeneration*

Degeneration related to aging is widespread, from cells to tissues to organs. The biological state of degeneration should be understood beyond the common knowledge of wear and tear. Prolonged or excessive use, like in the case of bones and joints, could be responsible for deterioration. However, other changes, either related to the innate biological make-up or to the molecular changes in response to environments, both internal and external, are as important. Nevertheless, whatever is the underlying cause, degeneration exists jointly with aging and remains the crucial factor in the patho-physiological changes.

1.1.3 *Decline in cell numbers*

Cells in the human body have proliferative capacity. With aging this capacity declines, the decline in proliferation not only brings about shrinkage in the volume, thence the normal function, but also affects the specialized functions which most collection of cells are responsible for.

The development of molecular biology has revealed that the interaction of cells leads to the production of specific proteins which are responsible for cell-to-cell interactions and some specific functions. Aging interferes with the normal production of normal proteins and brings about the production of abnormal proteins. Abnormal free radicals are also produced, the accumulation of which are responsible for further deterioration of cellular proliferation and their physiological function.

The abnormal proteins produced in response to aging might affect the normal cellular activities in another adverse direction. Complicated growth factors might be stimulated, leading to exaggerated proliferations i.e. the tendency of cancer growth (Sporn and Roberts, 1985).

1.1.4 *Changes in tissues and organs*

Both primary and secondary changes are observed. Firstly, aging affects the proliferation of stem cells which are responsible for the maintenance of different kinds of tissues. The decline in new batches of cells result in a decrease in the bulk of tissues and organs. The common occurrence of decreasing muscle bulk in the elderly and their residing jaws and sometimes even shrinking bone mass are good examples of stem cell deficiencies.

Secondary changes in the organs are observed when very often, with circulatory deterioration resulting in loss of tissue bulk, downgrading of function and even specific histo-pathological changes like fibrosis also occur. The most remarkable secondary effects are observed when endocrine glands are affected either directly via molecular influences, or indirectly through processes like declining circulation. Hormonal deficiencies thus resulted would have wide-spread implications in their target organs and functions.

The immunological system consists of a chain of cells, tissues and organs spread widely throughout the human body. Aging might have direct effect on any component of the organic chain, thus initiating the most complex immunological response, ranging from deficient functional activities which invite infections or cancer development; to over-activities which are responsible for allergic manifestations and perhaps autoimmune disorders.

Of all the tissue changes, those that are responsible for the most profound effects are the vascular changes which affect the effective blood-flow to tissues and organs. Without efficient blood flow, no proper function could be maintained.

1.2 Aging-Related Diseases

If cellular, tissue and organ changes simply lead to slowing down of physiological functions, aging could be taken as a normal process of life. Unfortunately, the aging related changes lead to diseases. There are four groups of diseases which closely follow aging:

(1) Cardiovascular changes
    Cholesterol deposits could be considered the culprit of cardiovascular diseases. The early degrees of endothelial thickening in arteries is responsible for hypertension. Affection of the coronaries would lead to coronary heart diseases and heart failure. Involvements of the carotid-cerebral distributions are leading to different forms of stroke.

(2) Musculo-skeletal decline
    The atrophying muscles, thinning cartilages, deforming joint surfaces, weakening tendons and ligaments, all lead to the decline of

biomechanical resilience and predispose to damages and injuries. Moreover, the pain associated depreciates the ability to maintain the normal locomotor activities, thus making aged people accident prone and injury susceptible.

(3) Neurological decline

The neurological deterioration takes a variety of changes that involve either a decrease in the number of functional cells or through disturbances of neuro-physiological activities via synapse communications or neurotransmitters. A panoramic manifestation thus may present as impaired memory, sleep disorders, judgement defects, dementias and problems of neuromuscular coordinations.

(4) Cancer development

Cells in specific sites are kept at a dynamic balance of apoptosis and proliferation for replacement. Under the influence of abnormal growth proteins, apoptosis is affected to different degrees. When the growth balance is thus affected, unchecked cellular proliferation provides the pathological basis of cancer development.

1.3 Healthy Aging

The concern with aging is obviously linked with the worry about diseases. One must realize that the groups of diseases just described as aging-related, are exactly those reported as top killers in affluent societies all over the world. The aging health problems have hence automatically emerged as public health foci of attention (German and Fried, 1989).

Public health authorities all over the world have, for many years, engaged in extensive propaganda, persuading people on nutritional issues like lowering cholesterol consumption, changing lifestyle, abstaining from smoking, and engaging in adequate physical exercises to maintain neuromuscular strength, etc.

Pharmaceuticals and food manufacturers, on the other hand, actively push new products into the consumer market, claiming extra nutritional values, yet devoid of harmful effects. The active consumer market has successfully misled the consumer that good health could be maintained, through the purchase of fancy new products, either in the form of drugs or special types of food.

Clinicians are aware of the expanding demand on health for the elderlies and special groups and clinics are organized to satisfy the need. Of all the active groups, one deserves special attention, *viz.* the "Anti-Aging Medicine Specialization" (AAMS) established recently in Europe and the US.[a] The following section will be dedicated to this new specialization and some details will be given since no other organization would be more representative that AAMS on the sophisticated efforts given to the clinical care of the elderly.

1.3.1 *Anti-aging medicine specialization (AAMS)*

The areas of concern of AAMS include the following:

*   nutrition,
*   hormonal deficiencies,
*   physical activities,
*   psychological state, and
*   environment.

1.3.1.1 *Nutrition*

The concern about nutrition is not confined to the choice of food, but involves a broad inspection on the processes of digestion and absorption which might be the source of nutrition-digestion related problems, irrespective of the quality or quantity of food items consumed.

For the sake of general understanding, AAMS has attempted to classify food as those bad for health and good for health. Under the "bad" category: there are the milk products, sugar and unsprouted grains; alcoholic, and caffeine-related soft drinks. Under the "good" category: there are fruits, vegetables and animal proteins; water and vegetable soups (Werbuch, 1993).

On the digestive side, AAMS emphasizes food allergy as the cause of age-related problems like obesity, bowel problems and fatigue. We are all aware of acute allergic reactions to specific food items and proteins that we are not used to, and the presentations of acute abdomen with pain, diarrhea

---

[a]Anti-Aging Medicine Specialization, created in 2002. Fifth year program, October 2007, six-day seminar http://www.euromedicom.jp/society/past_events/en_AmmsWeb.pdf

and perhaps vomiting. What AAMS addresses here is not the acute clinical presentations but subacute or hidden effects of allergic reactions to food intake. Two foci of pathogenesis are postulated, *viz.* change of intestinal flora, very often initiated by an overgrowth of yeasts and direct inflammatory changes. The subclinical allergy thus induces inflammation in the guts, upsetting the normal function and contributing towards the symptoms of aging. The manifestation could be obesity, irritable bowel syndrome and evidences could be obtained through the demonstration of serological changes and increases in cytokines like TNFα (Papadakis and Targan, 2000).

One new phenomenon which has been observed is labeled as "leaky gut syndrome." The postulation is that problems in digestion and absorption affect the excretory system so that abnormal excretions are initiated in the kidney system leading to unnecessary excretions and unnecessary retentions (Epstein, 1996), which contribute towards aging syndromes.

Obesity is one of the manifestations of aging and could be the result of the subclinical allergic reactions. Actually, obesity has been such a serious problem among the elderlies such that in Europe, special obesity clinics for the management of food problems have been inviting a lot of attention (Gibson, 2006).

Another area observed to be the result of food allergy is related to the frequent experience of fatigue among the elderly. A new syndrome, "Chronic Fatigue Syndrome," has therefore been created (Lindstedt *et al.*, 2007). The consistent feeling of fatigue is assumed to be either due to deficiency in one or more of the essential nutritional substances or from an overclose in one or more of the toxic influences from food. The essential nutritional substances include the vitamins, essential minerals and amino-acids and the different hormones. The toxic influences come from chemicals, changing intestinal flora, subclinical infections and allergens.

The AAMS obviously is adopting a deductive principle and is making an assumption that all physical and physiological manifestations, like obesity and fatigue, have an underlying cause which needs to be defined, then the opportunity of cure could be offered.

If external factors like food items could be the culprit of adverse physiological changes, the reactive results could be demonstrable either directly or indirectly through changes in the endocrine system.

1.3.1.2 *Hormonal problems*

Hormonal problems have been other targets of concern of the AAMS. Aging could be the cause of decline of activity of the endocrine systems, thus causing deficiencies. As a result of inflammation and allergy, endocrine systems could be adversely affected and deranged. The AAMS is therefore sensitive about the changes. Conventional clinical medicine is aware of major changes of excessive or deficient hormonal production which would be detected in the conventional laboratory tests. Subclinical changes emphasized by the AAMS experts, however, involve minor changes which are either ignored in the past or, using the conventional laboratory tools, are undetectable. AAMS has since establishment, invested tremendously on the creation of highly sophisticated laboratory tests catered towards the detection of minor alternations in hormonal levels, toxic material indicators, and apparently unimportant biochemical elements which have escaped clinician's attention in the past. Special laboratories capable of detecting those objective data are established to serve special services. The list of tests recommended by one of the newly established laboratories is given as an example (Table 1.1).

Table 1.1. Integrative functional medicine test menu (Metametrix Clinical Lab, Updated).

Symptoms/diseases	Tests
Metabolic syndrome	Metabolic Syndrome Profiles
Cardiovascular diseases	Cardiovascular Health Profiles, ADMA, CMP Test, Adrenal Stress; or +CoQ10, Fatty Acids, Lipid Peroxide
Obesity	Organix, Metabolic Syndrome, Cardiovascular Health Profiles
Diabetes	Metabolic Syndrome Profiles
Fatigue	Organix, Amino Acids, Triad, ION, Adrenal Stress
Chronic pain	Organix, Amino Acids; +GI fx (if gut pain), +Food Allergy, GI fx (if arthritis pain), +Minerals, Heavy Metals (if muscle pain), +Minerals, GI Fx (if cancer pain)
GI disorder	GI Fx
Liver disease, NOS	Organix, Amino Acids
Fatty liver	Organix, Fatty Acids
Chronic hepatitis B	Organix, Amino Acids, Nutrients and Toxic Elements
Cancer	Organix, ION, Estronex

Hormonal changes at micro levels are not provided by conventional laboratory hardwares and the nature of the "detectables" are specific to the particular system of concern. Since endocrine systems are complex and divergent, the attending clinician and his client have to sort out the area of concern before subjecting the investigation samples for testing (Table 1.2). The main systems of endocrine function include the thyroid, the adrenals and the gonadal systems. Patients' own active instructions on the major area of suspected problems, therefore, would be of utmost importance (Krabbe *et al.*, 2004).

1.3.2 *Comments on the deductive approach*

A review of the AAMS practice clearly revealed that aging is taken as a specific patho-physiological problem. Using scientific means to deal with this specific problem, therefore, requires the identification of the etiology, and then correction of what is apparently pathological. The deduction-ist believes that every phenomenon has a cause and unless the damage has been overwhelming and irreversible, otherwise, removal of the cause would offer an excellent opportunity of return to the normal. All is well if the aging problem is really the result of simple, straightforward "off-tracking" of normal physiological processes. Nevertheless, if aging is involving a multitude of declining physiological events subsequently turning pathological, targeting at single problems like "toxicity" or "deficiency" in specific areas might be able to give partial, temporary solutions only.

The success of modern science and clinical medicine in the past century has laid down a perfect background for the pursuit of the deductive solution to aging which, in specific cases, should be able to offer excellent results. The early successes must have laid down a good foundation for the establishment of more and more aging clinics. However, if the multitude of specific clinical tests fail to reveal the cause, no relevant treatment yet could be administered.

1.4 Aging in the Oriental Context

While aging has attracted the wide attention of clinicians and the public at large only after the awareness of the "senior boom," aging and longevity

Table 1.2. Specific groups of tests recommended for different clinical presentations.

Integrated Profiles	AccuChem Chlorinated Pesticides Profile
ION (Individual • Optimal • Nutrition) Profiles — blood and urine	AccuChem Volatile Solvents Profile
ION Pediatric — blood and urine	*Element Profiles*
Cardio/ION Profile — blood and urine	Nutrient and Toxic Elements — hair
TRIAD Profile — blood and urine	Nutrient and Toxic Elements — erythrocytes
TRIAD Bloodspot Profile	Toxic Metals — whole blood
Women's Health Profile — blood and urine	Nutrient and Toxic Elements 6–8 Hr — urine
Organix Profiles	Toxic Elements 6–8 Hr — urine
Organix Comprehensive — urine	Nutrient and Toxic Elements 24 Hr — urine
Organix Basic — urine	Toxic Elements 24 Hr — urine
Organix Dysbiosis — urine	
GI Effects Stool	*Health Risk Profiles*
GI Effects — stool analysis	ADMA (Asymmetric Dimethylarginine) — plasma
Amino Acid Profiles	Bone Resorption Assay — urine
Amino Acids 40 — plasma	Estronex 2/16 OH Ratio — urine
Amino Acids 20 — plasma	Metabolic Syndrome — serum and plasma
Amino Acids 40 — urine	Neopterin/Biopterin Profile — urine
Amino Acids 11 — blood spot	
Amino Acids 20 — blood spot	*Fat-Soluble Vitamin Profiles*
Homocysteine — plasma	Vitamin K Assay — serum
	Vitamin D Assay — serum
Fatty Acid Profiles	CoQ10 + Vitamin Profile — serum
Fatty Acid — plasma	Coenzyme Q10 — serum
Fatty Acids — erythrocytes	Fat-Soluble Vitamins Profile — serum
AA/EPA Ratio — plasma	
Fatty Acids — blood spot	*Oxidative Stress Indicators*
	Lipid Peroxides — serum
Allergix Profiles	DNA/Oxidative Stress Marker — urine
IgE Food Antibodies 30 — serum	
IgE Inhalant Antibodies — serum	*Hormone Profiles*
IgG4 Food Antibodies 90 — serum	Adrenal Stress Plus — saliva
IgG4 Food Antibodies — bloodspot 30	Adrenal Stress — saliva
Celiac Profile — serum	Insulin — serum
	IGF-1 — serum
Toxic Effects Profiles	Male Hormones — serum
Porphyrins Profile — urine	
AccuChem PCBs Profile — whole blood	

has always been a subject of public concern in the Oriental, particularly in the Chinese Society. Longevity is considered a wonderful gift of human fortune. Pursue of longevity draws no strict cut-off lines. All respected individuals, within the family, within the community and at a stage when personal successes are reaching remarkable levels, would start wishing to reach longevity. There should be no surprise therefore, that the practice of healthy survival starts long before what we currently realize as "elderly" or "geriatric" age.

The main philosophy in clinical practice is the prevention of falling sick, which is considered the backbone of Chinese medical practice. Herbs used in traditional Chinese Medicine, indeed, are categorized into three levels: the superior level herbs are used for prevention; the middle level are for early intervention; while the inferior level are for the actual treatment (which might be already too late).

Actually, the philosophy in clinical practice is guided by a broader philosophy of harmonization within the individual and harmonization of the individual with the outside world and with Heavenly Esteem. Chinese philosopher believe that the individual, in his pursue for knowledge and well-being, needs to make unlimited efforts of reasoning and attempts to bring himself to a higher spiritual level of existence. At the end, no matter which level he is capable of reaching, he well fulfils his duty and will be rewarded with satisfaction (Lewg and Lewg, 2006). Hence, good health in the Chinese philosophical context, is a state of holistic equilibrium in the physiological and physical activities. He has to at the same time, maintain the harmony with the outside Environment and with Society.

The principles of balanced nutrition would mean a regular consumption of simple food according to need (i.e. never overeat), choice of a balanced diet devoid of rich (fatty) varieties, and a clever choice of vegetable items which possess both nutritional as well as health promotion value.

1.5 The Concept of Herbal Intake to Support Aging

Longevity is a very much adored blessing. The well-known stories about how the Qin Emperor sent explorers outward from the "Middle Kingdom" in search for longevity herbs and how the Roman emperor Neru did the same were probably unique and genuine. In fact, with few exceptions elderly people value longevity as energetically.

Maintenance of health to reach longevity must be one of the most frequently pursued health practices that started ever since the beginning of human history, when the human mind became capable of positively manipulating events in life to bring better well-being. There is no need for special efforts to sustain this simple wish and remarkable folk practices on this direction have been sustained. Folk practice may have components of superstitious practices, which are finding difficulties to gain support in the scientific world. Herbal remedies on the other hand, are simple and straightforward, often giving gustatory pleasure on consumption, therefore maintaining its perpetuating popularity in Oriental communities. Western societies, on the other hand, particularly in the past century, are more indoctrinated to target-orientated specific treatment. Longevity appears too vague and broad in the scientific community.

A look at the development of modern pharmaceuticals would help understanding this phenomenon.

Europe was the focus of drug development in the 19th Century. Out of the different Europeans states, Germany has the strongest tradition of using medicinal herbs. Before the discovery of complicated pathologies of the human body, the traditional use of herbs and chemicals in the control of symptoms or symptom complexes formed the major direction of therapy. There was not much demand on scientific evidence. Prescription of herbs relied on experience, past or present.

Sometimes, frustrations on the uncertain outcome became so intense that a drastic and perhaps illogical approach developed, which was subsequently called homeopathic medicine. Homeopathic medicine advocates this working principle: since pathology was uncertain and the symptom complexes appeared so complicated, use a variety of modalities of medicinal herbs and/or chemicals with higher doses, to push for the maximal effects until adverse events appeared, then stop the treatment and treat the adverse effects. This illogical practice attracted followers and users, and to date, a small number of homeopathic hospitals are still active in different parts of Europe. Homeopathic medicine well illustrated the complexity of old clinical practices.

However, when the complicated pathological manifestations gradually became better explained, treatment shifted to more specific directions. At the same time, the rapid development of chemistry offered deeper levels of understanding between the chemical interactions after the drugs were administered. Chemists became excited when they identified direct chemical actions producing clinical relief. Some examples include: alkaline drinks neutralizing high acid contents, thus alleviating stomach aches; chemical laxatives producing gut mobility, thus causing bowel motion and effective treatment of constipation. More and more chemicals, and later biochemical explanations, were discovered in the enthusiastic pursuit for effective treatment chemicals. Pharmaceutical institutes were thence established to lead us into the victorious century of "bullet shot" treatment approach. The success of the pharmaceuticals naturally displaces the traditional unscientific services.

In Asia, on the other hand, the Industrial Revolution did not produce any direct change. It influence from Europe came later, and gradually. Folk medicine in India and China continued to enjoy unfading popularity. Single target identification and treatment using the magic bullet shot, no doubt, has been a great success in medicine and has solved numerous problems. However, when, instead of a single target, a disease entity is the result of complex changes involving many targets, the magic bullet would not work. Longevity involves complicated changes in the overall mechanisms of physiological aging, in which the magic bullet finds little application. One observes and speculates therefore that traditional medicine like Ayurveda in India and Chinese Medicine in China, would remain useful and important for aging.

Popularity could be maintained by just tradition. When no better way has yet emerged, tradition will enjoy more sustenance. When new scientific research methods and concepts appear and are applied to support the traditional approach, the traditional practice will be injected and replaced with modified approaches.

Whether this could be the current situation with traditional medicine could be verified with the attitude of some of the drug discoveries. Drug-development strategies have been influenced profoundly by the wealth of potential targets offered by genome projects. At present, the goal is to: (i) find a target of suitable function; (ii) identify

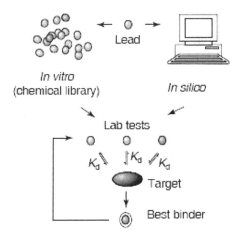

Fig. 1.2. Current drug development strategies.

the "best binder" by high-throughput screening of large combinatorial libraries and/or by rational drug design based on the three-dimensional structure of the target; (iii) provide a set of proof-of-principle experiments; and (iv) develop a technology platform that predicts potential clinical applications (Fig. 1.2). However, despite all the careful studies and the considerable drug-development efforts undertaken, the number of successful drugs and novel targets did not increase appreciably during the past decade. Furthermore, combinatorial therapy, which represents another form of multi-target drugs, is used increasingly to treat many types of diseases, such as AIDS, cancer and atherosclerosis (Csermely *et al.*, 2005). Snake and spider venoms are both multi-component systems and plants also employ batteries of various factors to fend off pathogenic attacks; thus, the use of multiple molecules is apparently evolutionary success story. Finally, traditional medical treatments often use multi-component extracts of natural products. Based on these examples and on our recent results of network analysis (Csermely *et al.*, 2005), it is proposed that systematic drug-design strategies should be directed against multiple targets, and that this novel drug-design paradigm might often result in the development of more-efficient molecules than the currently favored single-target drugs.

Development of a multi-target drug is likely to produce a drug that interacts with lower affinity than a single-target drug because it is unlikely that a small, drug-like molecule will bind to a variety of different targets with equally high affinity. However, low-affinity drug binding is apparently not a disadvantage. For example, meantime (a drug use to treat Alzheimer's disease) and other low affinity multi-target non-competitive NMDA receptor antagonists shows that low-affinity, multi-target drugs might have a lower prevalence and a reduced range of side-effects than high-affinity, single-target drugs (Csermely *et al.*, 2005).

1.6 Use of Chinese Herbs for Prevention of Aging-Related Disease

Herbs that have been observed to be suitable for keeping a holistic balance have been chosen as agents for disease prevention. These items are commonly used as vegetables in daily meals, either as a main dish or as components or ingredients. Examples are given in Table 1.3.

Some items within the same group of herbs have been used under more obvious pathological situations, either singly or in combination with other herbs. Examples are given in Table 1.4.

Table 1.3. Nutritional items favored in Chinese medicine.

人參	*Radix Ginseng*
黨參	*Radix Codonopsis*
黃芪	*Radix Astragali*
山藥	*Rhizoma Dioscoreae*
山楂	*Fructus Crataegi*
山奈	*Rhizoma Kaempferiae*
枸杞子	*Fructus Lycii*
沙參	*Adenophora stricta Miq.*
玉竹	*Rhizoma Polygonati Odorati*
百合	*Bulbus Lilii*
薏苡仁	*Semen Coicis*
蓮子	*Semen Nelumbinis*
黑芝麻	*Semen Sesami Nigrum*
冬蟲夏草	*Cordyceps*

Table 1.4. Anti-aging herbal items favored in Chinese medicine.

General (those used in food):	人參	*Radix Ginseng*
	黨參	*Radix Codonopsis*
	山藥	*Rhizoma Dioscoreae*
	蓮子	*Semen Nelumbinis*
	玉竹	*Rhizoma Polygonati Odorati*
	百合	*Bulbus Lilii*
	薏苡仁	*Semen Coicis*
	黑芝麻	*Semen Sesami Nigrum*
Supplementing hemopoiesis:	當歸	*Angelica sinensis*
	何首烏	*Radix Polygoni Multiflori*
	枸杞子	*Fructus Lycii*
	四君子湯	*Sijunzitang*
Supplementing Yin:	女貞子	*Fructus Ligustri Lucidi*
	玉竹	*Rhizoma Polygonati Odorati*
	桑椹	*Fructus Mori*
	四物湯	*Siwutang*
Supplementing Yang:	杜仲	*Cortex Eucommiae*
	鹿茸	*Cornu Cervi Pantotrichum*
	淫羊藿	*Herba Epimedu*
	腎氣丸	*Shenqiwan*

What are the clinical basis behind these herbs when they are used as preventive or treatment items? Do the items carry specific therapeutic effects? Or are they just used as "harmonizing" agents? And what does "harmonizing" mean in the modern clinical concept?

While research attempts are plentiful along the line of identifying specific therapeutic effects on specific herbal items, we have yet to wait for trustworthy evidences. Before that day, the simplest explanation given on the health value of the herbs could be their abilities to maintain an internal balance through the boostering up of an adequate state of immunological defense.

1.7 Function of Herbs Used for Longevity and Aging Diseases

The two most likely areas on which herbs may work to maintain health and prevention of aging-related diseases are immunomodulation and inflammation control. The former is related to self-defense and inflammation is the culprit of cellular and tissue degeneration.

In the past years, herbal items have been identified to be supportive of immunological defense. In the author's institute, mushroom extracts Gonoderma and Coriolus have been put through laboratory and clinical tests, results of which have well demonstrated the immunomodulating effects on normal individuals and patients suffering from nasopharyngeal carcinoma.

A summary of the two studies are supplied as follows:

1.7.1 *Example of upgrading immunological defense*

1.7.1.1 *Herbal formula as preventive agent to boost immunodefense*

Effect of Coriolus and Salvia on immunological function in healthy subjects:

- Design: placebo-controlled cross-over
- Primary objective: immunology marker
- Secondary objective: adverse effect
- Clients: two groups, Coriolus and Salvia + Placebo vs. Placebo + Coriolus and Salvia
- Treatment period: ten months (two months washout period included)
- Follow-up: every two months
- Results
  - up-regulates immune system
    - increases T helper cells
    - increases T suppressor cells

- increases T helper/T suppressor ratio
- increases B lymph cell
- increases quality of life
- increases vitality
- no adverse effects on liver and kidney

1.7.2 *Example of upgrading immunological defense to combat cancer*

Herbal formula (Coriolus and Salvia) as supplementary agent for patients suffering from nasopharyngeal carcinoma.

Results:

(1) fatigue was significantly improved in the supplement group;
(2) the immune markers decrease with radiotherapy in both the supplement and placebo groups, but the suppression of T lymphocytes percentage was significantly less in the supplement group than in the placebo group; and
(3) there was a general trend of deterioration of QoL scores after commencement of radiotherapy, not reaching statistical significant difference between the two groups.

It must be pointed out that many immuno-modulating herbs, depending on the dosage and the special circumstances, could be both up-regulating and down-regulating. An example is given in Fig. 1.3 which shows the clinical effects of an anti-allergic herbal formula in the control of allergic rhinitis. The effectiveness of the herbal formula in the situation of allergy illustrates its suppressive effects on the over-active immunological activities in allergic conditions.

In this clinical study of immunosuppression, when the herbal intake was discontinued, there was obvious sustained effects (which was not observed in the placebo group).

Allergic rhinitis — visual analog scale improvement.

1.8 Physical Activities

Adequate physical activities are advocated in both Western and Oriental communities as important elements to maintain healthy aging. However,

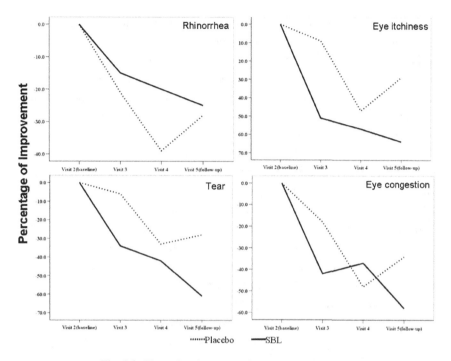

Fig. 1.3. Example of downgrading allergic responses.

while Western interpretation and practice of physical activities might refer to heavy exercises — competitive ball games, competitions and gymnastics which rely on plenty of energy consumption and sweating are popular in the West — Oriental exercises may take a different form of physical activities consisting of special stances, gentle movements, controlled breathing and meditation. Common practices of such Oriental exercises include *Taichi* and *Qigong* in China and yoga in India.

When such systems of meditation-exercise become more and more popular outside China and Asia, research aiming at the explanation of the activities is becoming more and more frequent. The National Institutes of Health in US has sponsored in 2007, a research program looking at the immunological effects of *Taichi* on people between 59 and 86. It was found that the *Taichi* group, compared to the Health Education group, enjoyed a 40% increase in immunological response to chickenpox vaccine. The rate of response was two times faster and there was also improved physical state, vitality and mental health (Irwin *et al.*, 2007).

Taichi can be and has been modified and utilized in different practical setting. In Japan, Sensei Jun Konno has pioneered a *Taichi* Training in the swimming pool. Participants work either singly, or preferably in a group. They stand on foot with body and shoulders immersed below water. With legs firmly stood and upper limbs free, some basic *Taichi* movements are slowly and forcibly performed under water. The body remain still and balanced.

What is being stressed is that physical activities involved, may be slow, however, well performed *Taichi* movements starts with good firm balance, and the stability of the mind is equally stressed. The practicing individual is required to meditate and keep the mental state at a most relaxed, undisturbed level. In the meantime, the slow movements allow deep, controlled breathing which is also essential for the relaxation of the mind. This *Taichi*, practiced in the water pool is called *Ai-Chi* in Japanese, and it has already attracted international attractions and different Ai-Chi clubs are being formed all over the world (Verhagen *et al.*, 2004).

The messages given to the early participants include:

(1) As we age, our sight, hearing, muscle strength, coordination and reflexes change, weakening our balance and leading to falls.

(2) Five percent of all falls result in serious injuries. However, even those not seriously affected suffer from psychological influences, which lead to impaired mobility, loss of function and an overall decline in the quality of life.

(3) One in three persons over 65, and one in two over 80 will fall at least once a year. These individuals would need special attention and awareness. Foot problems arising from deforming toes, arthritis and bad foot wears enhance the loss of balance.

(4) As we age, our sight, hearing, muscle strength, coordination and reflexes deteriorate, further weakening our balance. Co-existing medical diseases: cardiovascular, respiratory and diabetes, are other unwanted culprits.

(5) Since land exercises like "Rope Walk," "Balanced Stand," "Sit and Stand" are all simple and useful exercises good for maintaining the physical state of health, such modalities might appear bore when practiced in a long run. Moreover, such basic physical requirements have no meditation component.

Falling with or without injuries is disastrous for the elderly people. For those with fractures, apart from the prolonged healing, longevity is affected. For those without serious injury, it still means proneness to fall, impaired balance and possible decline in physical ability. Among the elderly, some are more prone to falls while some are not. This is of course related to their general physique and might be particularly related to their balancing ability. Scientific groups have tried various assessment means to detect those more prone to fall with the intension of providing them more serious training.

Assessing elderly people for their proneness to fall could be complicated because there are so many influencing factors, ranging from the internal pathology of the particular individuals to external environmental risks. The commonly adopted simple assessments: testing general muscle strength (grip), balance (timed stand) and endurance (six meter walk) are useful means to get some basic idea about an elderly person's physical ability, and hence, his ability to resist falls. The test results would hardly indicate the individual's absolute state of physical well-being, but the results taken, when compared with similar tests performed some months' earlier and later, will be useful objective indicators of change.

1.9 Living in Harmony

Ancient philosophers in China and India emphasized a lot on living in harmony within the community and with nature. Meditation is a way to maintain one's internal harmony from which the individual also reaches out for harmony with community and nature.

There was the famous Okinawa Centenarian Research done by Nobuyoshi Hirose. Hirose wanted to know why the Okinawa people enjoy such a healthy longevity as there were so many centenarians. He found that the Okinawa people ate a healthy diet with a lot of fish and vitamins. They had plenty of exercises, plenty of sleep and little stress. With regard to the environment, the islands provided fresh air, fresh water, adequate sunshine, peaceful and green surroundings and simple but convenient medical facilities. On the social side, people lived good community life and enjoyed recreations. Using modern medical terms common in research planning, the centenarians enjoyed excellent quality of life.

Harmony in the broadest sense: internal, social, environmental and ecological; therefore, it is the goal to pursue in the quest for healthy aging.

In the modern affluent society, the scientific approach is the norm in the past 100 years. The individual patient is taken as the living organism assumingly having the identical structures and biological functions. Sickness is taken as a straightforward structural or functional change which is usually correctable, unless the discovery is too late or the individual too old. This is the scientific concept behind "target" treatment. It works very well if the cause of sickness is really uniform and focused. Nevertheless, it has been observed in the recent decade that diseases are in fact more complicated. The cause of a disease could be related to multiple causes and interactions between many dysfunctions. Treatment, therefore, becomes much more difficult and results more uncertain.

When removal of a single pathology becomes a myth and multiple pathologies are not removable, the concept of maintaining the balance becomes important. Likewise, prevention becomes more important. The need to be more concerned with the individual's genomic make-up, psychological state, personal habits, social behaviour and environmental situations become important for the maintenance of harmony.

1.10 The Real Situation That We Are Facing

If we start to feel the decline with aging and experience flailty we will be facing a real dilemma today when we consider getting the benefits from available medications or supplements. Shall we rely totally on clinical investigations through the help of various specialists, or shall we just go to the drug store or supermarket to shop for the best packed items recommended by friends and neighbours or in the media?

Specialists keen to advise on medication include the cardiologist, the osteoporosis expert (endocrinologist, geriatrician, gynecologist) and the family physician. These experts have excellent information about target orientated drugs with specific aim, e.g. on the lowering hypertension, cholesterol level; improving bone mineral density etc. The effectiveness of the specific drugs is based on high quality clinical trials which relied on biostatistics analysis.

When the purpose of receiving the drug(s) is for longevity and prevention of diseases, do we really need the "most thorough" treatment? The grey area across "established problem" and "potential problem" is wide, sometimes changing, because physiological data do change with time.

The situation of health supplement is no better. Pharmaceuticals are recommended by specialists and the scientific evidences and efficacy are considered universally reliable. The health supplements have not gone through scientific evaluation and therefore does not possess objective data of efficacy. Spectacular advertisements have comfortably taken over the job of promotion. People feel tempted to try new preparations with new promises.

When everyone runs after healthy aging, there is plenty of room for sophisticated machines to convince users that minor or micro-deviations from normal ranges are abnormal and deserve treatment. There are also plenty of buyers of health supplements which claim efficacies in various areas of concern. A new term has since been created: "medicalization." Diversions from the normal ranges have been medicalized. Ordinary food and drink have been medicalized. It would be a good policy for everyone to take good care of himself or herself to promote good health and prevent diseases, whether having an inclination towards Western or Oriental approach. In so doing, everyone needs to avoid being the victim of medicalization.

References

Buckwalter, J.A., Heckman, J.S. and Petrie, D.P. (2003) Aging of the North American population: New challenges for orthopaedics. *J. Bone Joint. Surg.* **85A**(4), 748–758.

Csermely, P., Ágoston, V. and Pongor, S. (2005) The efficiency of multi-target drugs: The network approach might help drug design. *Trends Pharmacol. Sci.* **26**, 178–182.

Epstein, M. (1996) Aging and the kidney. *J. Am. Soc. Nephrol.* **7**, 1106–1122.

German, P.S. and Fried, L.P. (1989) Prevention and the elderly: public health issues and strategies. *Annu. Rev. Public Health* **10**, 319–332.

Gibson, E.L. (2006) Emotional influences on good choice: Sensory, physiological and psychological pathways. *Physiol. Behav.* **89**(1), 53–61.

Irwin, M.R., Olmstead, R. and Oxman, M.N. (2007) Augmenting immune responses to varicella zoster virus in older adults: A randomized controlled trial of Tai Chi. *J. Am. Geriatr. Soc.* **55**(4), 511–517.

Krabbe, K.S., Petersen, M. and Bruunsgaard, H. (2004) Inflammatory mediators in the elderly. *Exp. Gerontol.* **39**(5), 687–699.

Lewg, Z.M. and Lewg, S.C. (2006) *Anti-Ageing Herbs*. Natural Health Press, Hong Kong (in Chinese).

Lindstedt, G., Eggerstern, R. and Sunbeck, G. (2007) Thyroid dysfunction and chronic fatigue. *Lancet* **358**, 151.

Papadakis, K.A. and Targan, S.R. (2000) Role of cytokines in the pathogenesis of inflammatory bowel disease. *Annu. Rev. Med.* **51**, 289–298.

Sporn, M.B. and Roberts, A.B. (28 February 1985) Autocrine growth factors and cancer. *Nature* **313**, 745–747.

Verhagen, A.P., Immink, M., van der Meulen, A. and Bierma-Zeinstra, S.M. (2004) The efficacy of Tai Chi Chuan in older adults: a systematic review. *Fam. Pract.* **21**(1), 107–113.

Werbuch, M.R. (1993) *Nutritional Influences on Illness*. Third Line Press, Taszana, CA (ISBN: 09618550-3-7).

Chapter 2

Study on Thoughts of "Treating Disease Before Its Onset" from Famous CM Doctors

Chun-Bo Xu and Xiang-Yong Zhang

Abstract

The thoughts of "Treating Disease before Its Onset" has been valued, enriched and developed by generations of CM doctors to be a major theory guiding daily health care, disease prevention and treatment in TCM systems. In this new century, as the public opinion of healthcare and medical mode transforms and with the advent of global crisis in medical care, the National Outline for Medium- and Long-Term Science and Technology Development states that "with an emphasis on prevention, more effort should be put in the prevention and treatment of diseases to integrate health promotion and disease prophylaxis and treatment." According to this outline, the focus of medical care should shift from disease treatment to prophylaxis. In November 2007, the "CM Treating Disease before Its Onset Project" was initiated and its underlying theory is drawing ever-increasing attention. This article, by analyzing the idea of "Treating Disease before Its Onset," aims to discuss the inheritance and carrying forward of experiences from famous CM doctors, so as to popularize the thought and promote public health conditions.

Keywords: Traditional Chinese Medicine (TCM); Prevention of Diseases; Health Maintenance; Longevity; Lifestyle; Age-Related Disease; Body Resistance.

2.1 The Origins of the Thoughts of "Treating Disease Before Its Onset"

The goals of medicine are not simply to cure diseases, but rather to prevent them. Ever since the very beginning of CM, doctors have realized the importance of preventing diseases. As discussed in different chapters of *Huang Di Nei Jing*, such as *Su Wen·Si Qi Tiao Shen Lun Pian, Su Wen·Ba Zheng Shen Ming Pian, Su Wen·Ci Re Pian,* and *Ling Shu·Ni Shun,* "The sages did not treat those already ill, but treated those not yet ill"; "The good doctors treated the disease in the bud before its outbreak"; "Although the symptoms are not seen yet, give acupuncture to patients with a reddish color on their faces (to prevent the disease from developing). This is called Treating Disease before Its Onset"; "The good doctors treated patients whose diseases had yet to develop," the idea of "Treating Disease before Its Onset" is explained in *Huang Di Nei Jing* in two aspects, prevention of diseases and containment of diseases to avoid any unexpected changes. CM doctors of later times inherited and further developed this idea.

The concept of "Treating Disease Before Its Onset" was elaborated in *Nan Jing* in a perspective of controlling progression of diseases from one organ to another by stating that "knowing liver affects spleen, if liver disease is diagnosed, the spleen *qi* shall be consolidated to prevent liver pathogens from spreading to spleen, and this is called treating disease before its onset."

Zhang Zhongjing during the Han dynasty suggested many specific measures in the context of health preservation and disease prevention, early treatment after disease onset, progression and transformation control, and prevention of disease relapse, as applications of the "Treating Disease before Its Onset" theory. In *Jin Kui Yao Lue* he wrote: "if men can take good care of themselves without their meridians and collaterals being interfered by pathological wind; even if interfered, treat in time the diseases before they progress to organs; even if organs affected, use a series of treatment to avoid the obstructions of the nine orifices, in addition, do not bleach laws or get injured by animals, have controlled sex, have all variety of food, and have no decline in their body functions, there is no way diseases can invade the skin and subcutaneous tissues."

Sun Simiao during the Tang Dynasty pointed out that "people who cultivate their characters treat diseases before their outbreak." He also created a set of methods that promote longevity. By categorizing diseases into three phases: diseases long before onset; diseases immediate before onset; and diseases that already broke out, he emphasized that good doctors would treat diseases before their onset and the exhibition of any symptoms.

Zhu Danxi during the Jin-Yuan era suggested it was better off to take care of health when there is no disease than treating them after outbreaks. His focus was the early prevention and treatment of diseases. Other doctors suggested moxa-moxibustion for prevention of diseases together with other health-care methods.

Ye Tianshi during the Qing Dynasty highlighted the importance of "reinforcement of unaffected areas," and, according to patients' conditions, took different measurements to control progression of febrile diseases. Wu Jutong in his *Wen Bing Tiao Bian* suggested preservation of fluid and prevention of *yin* damage methods of treating febrile diseases, which also implied the underlying concept of "Treating Disease before Its Onset."

Diseases before their onset, as referred to by CM doctors in history, actually include three stages: disease before onset; disease after outbreak; and disease after being cured. The soul of "Treating Disease before Its Onset" thought is to prevent diseases from happening, prevent progression if the diseases have already broken out, and prevent relapse after recovery. There are other people who further divided it into four stages: long before onset; immediately before onset; after disease outbreak; and after recovery. They advocate health care in daily life; prevention of diseases before onset; treating of diseases when patients are about to get ill to prevent disease progression; in case diseases already break out, treat disease as soon as possible; and nourishing patients' body after diseases to avoid relapses.

Prevention of disease before onset mainly refers the soothing of mental conditions, strengthening of resistance to prevent diseases from happening. It reflects the CM health care thought of "nourishing out body when no diseases have surfaced." The ideal is for human beings to live a disease-free life of high quality.

Prevention of disease progression when it already breaks out has two meanings: first being the prevention of disease development when it is just initiated, and secondly the early treatment to prevent disease from progressing and transforming after it is initiated. When diseases are about to break out, early treatment is necessary for preventing them from developing and eliminating them as they are not yet severe. However, when diseases have already broken out, active control of disease progression needs to be taken in order to treat it.

Prevention of relapses after recovery means to take extra care in health maintenance immediately after patients recover from diseases so as to prevent the recurrence of the diseases. Patients who are newly recovering from diseases usually have deficiency in vital *qi*, disorder of *qi* and blood, and imbalance between *yin* and *yang*. If not taken good care of, it is very common to have diseases relapse in these patients and it is a waste of previous therapeutic efforts.

2.2 The Thought of "Treating Disease Before Its Onset" from Famous CM Doctors

Famous CM experts are clinically experienced and academically of high attainments, representing the highest level of current development of CM both academically and clinically. They have inherited from the ancient CM physicians the "Treating Disease before Its Onset" thought, and further developed it.

2.2.1 *Emphasizing on physical and mental health preservation; valuing the balance between exercise and resting; using nourishing food rather than medicines as restoratives and depending on different situations, use accordingly*

Many of famous CM doctors thoroughly understand ways of health care and live long lives. They stress on a moderate diet, a regular daily schedule, and enough rest. Their knowledge in health care is worth referred to for the public as guidance in daily life.

Zha Yuming, at an age over 90, was still able to see and hear clearly, think logically, and talk sonorously. When asked by patients of any tips, his answers are to: "have a balanced diet of whole and refined grains in daily three meals; drink frequently green teas and say no to tobacco and alcohol; take a walk after meals and strengthen spleen and stomach functions; keep early hours to be energetic; build up physique, exercise waist and pound in back; have less desires and conserve energy; do not be angry and that is beneficial to heart and lung; take a nap for a while to remove exhaustion; keep hands and brains busy so they do not functionally degenerate; if u adhere to these, you can expect to live a hundred years." Mr. Zha believes a carefree and peaceful mental condition, as well as having less desires and being confident and lenient to others, are key to longevity, and the core of preserving health.

Gan Zuwang, at an age over 90, was still full of vigor. His tip was to "think like a child, eat like an ant, crave like a turtle, and act like a monkey." In other words, he suggests to keep heart young and carefree, have a balanced and moderate diet, be open-minded and magnanimous, and exercise often.

Taking nourishing food and/or tonics to preserve health should go according to certain rules such as food shall be given first before tonics and different tonics should be used differently in different patients' situations. Yan Dexin points out that "nourishing food is better than tonics because the latter supplement the body unevenly and function as cures to diseases, thus they should not be taken indiscriminatively or in long term. However, some food items that we daily consume could nourish our body and treat diseases as well." This is in good accordance with what was stated in *Qian Jin Fang*, "to treat diseases, nourishing food shall be given first; only if this does not work should medications be used." Medications could be supplementing or reducing while our body could be deficient or excessive in certain functions. Only when the right method of reinforcing and reducing is used could desired effects be seen. However, people nowadays tend to use tonics indiscriminatively. Concerned by this, Mr. Zha stresses importance the appropriate use of tonics. Even precious tonics like ginseng and pilous antler, if misused, will lead to excessive functioning of organs and *yin-yang* disharmony, and become the cause of diseases. Therefore, taking tonics indiscriminatively without understanding the diseases should be avoided.

Fang Heqian points out that one cannot rely purely on tonics for strengthening of body resistance to consolidate constitution, but rather tonics should be used in combination with diet. A balanced combination will be beneficial in reinforcing stamina and *qi*. In terms of adverse effect of tonics, he believes that long term use of agents that reinforces *yang* will cause deficient fire and thus should be given with buffering agents that are soft and moisturizing. Agents that nourish *yin*, on the other hand, if used excessively, will affect stomach functions and shall be used in combination with drugs that recuperate stomach *qi*. The principle is to reinforce *qi* but not to alter the balance and to nourish *yin* but not to affect stomach functions.

2.2.2 *Grasp the trend of disease progression; put prevention as priority, control the origin, and truncate the progression*

There are certain rules for any development and progression of diseases. At the initial stage, diseases are easier to treat. As they progress, it becomes more difficult to cure them. Therefore, treating diseases at the beginning stage before any symptoms surface and starting prevention in young people to block and reverse the progression of diseases will effectively control disease development so as to prevent disease onset in the first place, and avoid aggravation of the diseases if they already are initiated.

(1) Prevention of serious diseases from developing ailments. Li Furen always says "serious diseases arise from ailment; chronic diseases arise from acute ones; diseases difficult to treat arise from those easily cured." He thinks the treatment of pulmonary diseases should start with prevention and treating exogenous fever. Good lifestyle habits should be maintained to eliminate chances of external pathogens invading our body. Treat in time exogenous fever to prevent it from progressing into tracheitis, pneumonia, and other pulmonary diseases. The key to prevent and treat chronic obstructive lung disease is to eliminate exogenous fever and acute bronchitis.

(2) Prevention of age-related disease at young age. Wang Mianzhi identifies cardiovascular diseases; hypertension and hyperlipidemia are severe threats to health conditions of aged people. As nutritional conditions improve, life and working paces change, affected population of such diseases is becoming younger. He thus proposes to "prevent and treat age-related diseases in youth and middle-aged". When dealing with these diseases, he emphasizes the importance of holism in bringing the recuperative effect of TCM into play to prevent disease progression to cardiovascular diseases, diabetes, encephalatrophy, cerebromalacia and stroke. Protection of heart, spleen, and kidney is also addressed. "Treating Disease Before Its Onset" concept underlies the overall treatment strategy.

(3) Diagnosis from subtle changes for early prevention and treatment. He Yanshen usually examines the tongue of patients with acute pulmonary heart diseases. It is a warning sign of pulmonary encephalopathy if the tip of the tongue is red in color or has dark red granules on

it. Hence, Cornu Rhinocerotis and other ingredients should be given added into the Decoction for Reliving Dryness of the Lung and given in combination with *Angong Niuhuang Wan*. He believes that timely treatment with above-mentioned medications in most cases can prevent the pulmonary encephalopathy from developing. Even if the disease breaks out, it is usually less severe in patients treated in time and full recovery is more common.

(4) Clearing lung heat in pneumonia in the elderly even heat has not surfaced. Li Furen considers pneumonia in the elderly different from ordinary pneumonia. It is non-typical in symptoms and easily progressed to induce a variety of organ failures and thus, it is thought to be a critical disease in the elderly. Ordinary pneumonia normally arises from exogenous fever that is resulted from pathogenic heat invasion into the interior from exterior. The reason for no typical heat seen in pneumonia in the elderly is the deficiency of vital *qi* and the resultant non-fierce competition between the vital *qi* and pathogenic factors. Therefore, besides diffusing and moisturizing the lung, clearing lung heat should also gain our attention in clinical context. The addition of ingredients that clear lungs, such as Cortex Mori, honeysuckle bud and flower, *Forsythia Suspensa*, Scutellaria, Heartleaf Houttuymia herb, and dandelion to the medication would be even better effective.

(5) The establishment of "Blocking and Reversing Therapy" in prevention and treatment of chronic severe hepatitis. Chronic severe hepatitis refers to the subacute hepatic necrosis based on chronic hepatitis or cirrhosis. It progresses rapidly and endangers patients' life. Having realized the specific pattern in its pathogenesis, transmission among organs, and conversion between deficiency and excess, Qian Ying established multiple "Blocking and Reversing Therapies." The "Pathology Blocking and Reversing Therapy" is based on the pathogenesis of the disease that progresses from toxic dampness-blood stasis-deficiency that is characterized by root deficiency and branch excess. Various methods are employed, including eliminating dampness to remove phlegm, clearing heat-toxin, soothing liver and regulating *qi*, promoting blood circulation for removing blood stasis, nourishing the kidney *yin*, and warmly invigorating spleen and kidney, in patients showing early pathogenic signs. "Organ-transmission Blocking and Reversing

Therapy" stresses the pattern of the disease transmitting among organs and treat the disease by severing the pathogens from transmission and strengthening vital *qi* according to the characteristics of liver diseases and other involved organs like spleen, stomach and kidney. "Blocking and Reversing Therapy in Different Stages of Disease Course" treats liver diseases differently based on the characteristics of the diseases at initial, intermediate, and late stages. At the early stage, methods for clearing and soothing the liver are adopted. Later at intermediate stage, coordinating of liver functions is of more importance. Finally, if the disease has already progressed to late stage, nourishing and emolliating of liver is the treatment strategy. Mr. Qian often uses *Qianjin Xijiao San* with addition of *Yinchenhao Tang* Oriental Wormwood Decoction as treatment for rapid blocking of the diseases. The reversing of the diseases, on the other hand, is usually facilitated by using high dose of *Astragalus Membranaceus*, Radix Aconti Lateralis Preparata, and cinnamon. All the above-mentioned therapeutic approaches emphasize on early treatment and truncate the progression of the disease to prevent its spreading to unaffected parts in patients, and they represent an innovative application of the long-held ideal that "the good doctors treat the disease in the bud before its outbreak."

2.2.3 *Adjust medication and dosage and choose the right time to treat disease according to the changes in patients' condition in the four seasons*

Humans are reflections of surrounding environments. The changes in physiological functions and pathological conditions are in correspondence to changes in the environments. Diseases are different in nature in the four seasons and the treatment should be adjusted accordingly.

Gan Zuwang thinks since the five sense organs are anatomically open to the environment and thus more prone to the influence from the external world, prevention and treatment of diseases should change accordingly with time. For instance, allergic rhinitis commonly breaks out in spring while atrophic rhinitis and laryngopharyngitis normally happens in autumn, therefore, in those two seasons great effort should be put in prevention of such diseases. In winter, rhinitis and nasal sinusitis patients who are deficient in kidney *yang* often have their disease aggravated. Therefore, Radix Aconti Lateralis Preparata, cinnamon, Rhizoma Zingiberis and asarum should be used for treatment. In summer, patients who have spleen *qi* deficiency show thickened tongue fur and filthy turbidity in secretion from ear and nose. In this situation, Agastache, Fortune Eupatorium herb, and lotus leaf are appropriate additions to treatment. The dosage of medications should be adjusted based on different seasons as well. For example, Radix Aconti Lateralis Preparata, cinnamon, and Rhizoma Zingiberis should be given with *Jinkui Shenqi Wan* in winter to treat patients with deficiency in *yang*. However, they should be given in a reduced dose or not given to patients in summer time.

Gan thinks wind in spring, heat in summer, dryness in autumn and coldness in winter could all have major impact on epistaxis, and should be treated differently. In spring, Schizonepeta Tenuifolia and Divaricate Saposhnikovia Root should be used to dispel wind and diffuse the lung; in summer, it should be Agastache, Fortune Eupatorium herb, and lotus leaf that are employed for clearance of summer heat and resolving dampness; in autumn, moisturizing dryness is the main aim. *Sang Xing* Decoction should be given for warm dryness while Decoction for Reliving Dryness of the Lung is used to treat cold dryness; in winter, removal of stasis should be focused on. For patients with heat, tree peony root bark, red peony root, and Rubiaceae are useful to cool the blood and promote circulation. For patients with deficient cold, Chinese Angelica, saffron, and pollen typhae are added to the treatment to warm and open meridians and collaterals.

2.2.4 *Value the strengthening of body resistance and preservation of stomach qi; rely on innate resistance to treat diseases*

CM believes that "if vital *qi* is sufficient in body, no invasion of pathological factors is possible". Treating disease is much more than simply removing pathological factors. It also requires the adjustment of the physiological functions of our body to re-establish balance between *yin* and yang so as to cure the diseases. Therefore, said Zhang Jingyue, "there is no one whose disease persists when the vital *qi* is restored, and vice versa, there is no one who do not fall ill when the vital *qi* is depleted."

(1) Strengthening body resistance to consolidate constitution. Strengthening body resistance means strengthening vital *qi* and tonifying *qi*, blood, *yin* and *yang*. Consolidating constitutions refers to reinforcement of spleen and kidney primordial *qi*. In sum, strengthening body resistance to consolidate constitution implies the restoration of organ functions from a perspective oh holism to promote body's resistance to diseases. There are many means to achieve this goal, namely medication, acupuncture and moxibustion, qigong, exercise, mental counseling, and balanced diet. Many famous CM doctors have discussed on this issue.

Fang Heqian recognizes strengthening of vital *qi* the key to treat diseases. Many diseases, especially severe diseases and internal injury and miscellaneous diseases at late stage, affect spleen and kidney functions. Hence, treatment will only be effective if it reinforces the spleen and kidney. Based on this understanding, Fang created the *Zibu* Decoction that strengthens *yin, yang, qi* and blood in spleen and kidney to reinforce the constitution and re-establish *yin-yang*, *qi* and blood balance. The formula of the *Zibu* Decoction is a representative of treatment dealing with organ deficiency and decline. By strengthening vital *qi* and consolidating the constitution, the *Zibu* Decoction is able to prevent the disease from progressing, as an application of the concept "Treating Disease before Its Onset."

The guideline He Ren advocates in treating cancers is to "continuously strengthen vital *qi*, attempt to remove the pathological factors at right timing, and adjust treatment with changed pathological conditions." He thinks the initiation and development of cancer is closely associated with deficiency in vital *qi* and insufficient resistance. As a result, he emphasizes the strengthening of vital *qi* as the basis, while trying to resist cancer growth at the right timing and adjust treatment with changes in disease state, in order to effectively improve patients' resistance, control disease development, prolong survival, or even fully recover.

Li Furen thinks it is more important to strengthen vital *qi* than removing pathological factors in elderly patients. Consequently, he usually adds in formulas such as resolving exterior, dispelling wind, clearing heat, removing phlegm, diffusing lung, regulating stomach, regulating the flow of *qi*, channeling, pacifying liver, promoting blood circulation, removing obstruction in collaterals, excreting dampness, relaxing bowels, and resolving masses that remove pathological factors *Lycium Chinense*, Radix Codonopsis, and Astragalus plant that function to strengthen vital *qi*. Sometimes, formulas that strengthen vital *qi* like *Yupingfeng* Power, *Danggui Buxue* Decoction, *Liuwei Dihuang* Decoction, and *Erzhi Wan* are included in the treatment to avoid damaging vital *qi* while removing pathological factors or even strengthening it while removing pathological factors.

(2) Preserving stomach *qi*. Spleen and stomach are the acquired foundation and provide the source of *qi* blood formation. Digestion and transportation of medication and food require the function of spleen and stomach. Once the spleen and stomach functions are impaired, not only is resistance weakened by insufficient source for *qi* blood formation, but medications cannot be transported to the sites of diseases as well. This is described as "no drug will exert effect if the stomach *qi* is depleted."

Professor Zhang Zhenyu thinks preserving stomach *qi* should be noted in treating exogenous pathological factors and internal damage. When treating exogenous wind fever, provided that pathological heat easily damages *yin*, Reed Rhizome is used to clear heat for promoting production of fluid, thus preserves stomach *yin*; if patients feel thirsty, is constipated, or showa red-colored tongue, Radix Rehmanniae and common Anemarrhena rhizome are used to clear heat and nourish *yin* to preserve stomach *qi*; at late stages of febrile diseases when excessive heat cannot be removed, use *Zhuye Shigao* Decoction to plainly reinforce *qi* and to promote production of fluids, as well as pacifying stomach. Zhang emphasizes that when treating internal damage, enhancing source for (*qi*-blood) formation should always accompany tonifying deficiency regardless of the site of disease. For example, use Chinese Angelica, *Danshen* root, and *Polygala tenuifolia* together with ginseng and tuchahoe to nourishing the heart; use *Liuwei Dihuang Wan* together with ginseng to nourish the kidney; principles of formulating treatment to nourish the lungs are based on earth generating metal; liver diseases are usually treated by soothing the liver and regulating *qi* as well as strengthening the spleen and regulating stomach functions.

Fang Heqian values "preservation of stomach *qi* and fluids." He suggests that "the priority in treating patients with deficiency in diseases", and that "spleen and stomach functions must be taken good care of in severe diseases." Ingredients that regulate the stomach, nourish *yin*, and benefit *qi* like Fried Fructus Setariae Germinatus, medicated leaven, radish seeds, Fructus Amomi, chicken gizzard-membrane, lily bulb, dwarf lilyturf tuber, fragrant Solomonseal Rhizome, *Caulis Dendrobii*, jujube, and *Radix et Rhizoma Glycyrrhizae* are often seen in his formulas. To treat deficiency caused by long-term diseases and elderly patients, Fang stresses the importance of "restoring stomach functions when disease is surfaced" and believes preservation of stomach *qi* can strengthen vital *qi* and remove pathological factors. But the administration of medication has to be gradual and the choice of drugs being balanced in nature. It is better for the dose to be low. Overall, treatment should be balanced, not being extreme in any directions so long-term use is harmless. The preservation of stomach *qi* enables proper functioning of spleen and stomach, soothing of lung *qi*, pacification of liver *qi*, reinforcement kidney *Qi*, so that all organs remain healthy.

Guo Ziguang emphasizes spleen and stomach protection in treating cancers. He recognizes that maintaining of proper functioning of spleen and stomach is the key in treating cancers, and one of the advantages of TCM in treating cancers. Only when spleen and stomach are functioning properly can they digest food as source for *qi*-blood formation, thus replenishing the loss of vital *qi* in coping with cancer. There are two ways of maintaining the proper functions of the spleen and stomach. Firstly, do not use drugs with high toxicity; be careful using drugs too hot or cold in nature; use less agents that nourish and cause spleen stasis. If these drugs are necessary, use them with agents that protect spleen and stomach or drugs that promote spleen functions. Secondly, use mainly methods that employ bland and sweet-natured drugs to reinforce the spleen, pungent and aromatic-natured drugs to promote stomach functions, and aromatic-natured drugs to promote spleen functions. A few formulas that follow this principle include *Shenling Baizhu* Powder, *Xiangsha Liujunzi* Decoction, *Zhaqu Pingwei* Powder, *Huoxia Pingwei* Powder, and *Jianpi Wan*.

Hu Jianhua proposes that "whichever organ is in diseased state, nourishing spleen and stomach is always suggested", in the belief that the initiation and progression of any diseases are always closely associated with spleen and stomach. In clinical context, this means the protection of spleen and stomach functions. More specifically, there are a few rules to follow: the nourishing of spleen *qi*, the nourishing of stomach *yin*, close monitoring of ascending and descending in spleen and stomach diseases, promotion of stomach function while reinforcing *qi* to treat diseases caused by consumptive deficiency, warming of the spleen and stomach to reinforce *yang* while avoiding damaging *yin*, and termination of treatment that clears pathological factors once disease has been controlled.

Qian Bowen stresses that nourishing spleen *qi* should be combined with nourishing stomach *yin* to avoid damaging one while reinforcing the other. He often uses snakeground root, dwarf lilyturf tuber, Radix Adenophorae, and *Caulis Dendrobii* in application of the principle he advocates. The dose of snakeground root is usually 30–60 g for patients who show fissured red tongue.

2.2.5 *Value the theory of interactions among organs and treat diseases in multiple organs at the same time to enrich the concept of "Treating Disease Before Its Onset"*

Human organs are interlinked with each other closely. The disease in one organ could progress to other organs by affecting upstream or downstream organs, or exterior-interior transmissions. Treating diseases in multiple organs often effectively control the progression of diseases.

In the context of spleen and stomach diseases, Li Zhenhua thinks treating diseases in the spleen and stomach have to be performed at the same time. Hence, drugs that promote spleen function should be used in treating stomach disease and vice versa. Lu Zhizheng thinks treatment of mid-retention caused by dampness needs to be approached from both spleen and stomach. That is to clear spleen dampness by promoting stomach functions using Fructus Amomi, Pericarpium citri reticulatae, Fructus Aurantii, and citron fruit peels; to eliminate stomach dampness by promoting spleen functions using Fortune Eupatorium herb, Agastache, cardamom, coix seed, and Indian bread, in an attempt to "reinforce and pacify the unaffected area before diseases progress to such places."

Promoting spleen functions and reinforcing spleen *qi* have been regular treatment in treating liver diseases since the long-suggested theory that
"liver diseases can cause spleen diseases and thus reinforced spleen function
is needed to prevent it from being affected by liver pathology." However, Qian
Ying believes merely nourishing spleen *qi* is not enough for chronic liver treatment and nourishing stomach *yin* is also recommended. This is because majority of liver diseases are caused by dampness-heat. Dampness weakens spleen
yang while heat weakens stomach *yin*. Therefore, if patients display dryness on
tongue and mouth or constipation, the treatment should include reinforcement
of spleen *qi* together with nourishing stomach *yin*. Moreover, Qian thinks as
chronic liver disease progresses, in most cases they result in deficiency in liver
and kidney *yin*. Since the liver and kidneys originate from the same source,
nourishing liver *yin* will cause the deficiency of the common source due to
competition. However, this could be solved by nourishing both the liver and
kidneys. Therefore, Qian proposes that "the origin of liver diseases lies in kidney and reinforcement of kidney *qi* is the priority." By stressing treating liver
diseases by nourishing the kidneys and nourishing the kidneys as a measure
of protecting liver, Qian becomes the first in history of CM practitioners to
establish such relationship between the liver and kidneys.

Liu Bichen puts forward that treating nephritic syndrome in children
should start from the lung. Liu thinks the disease is closely associated
with the invasion of exogenous pathological factors. In the early phase,
it commonly comes in conjunction with symptoms normally occurring in
lung-related diseases such as runny nose, cough, fever, and sore throat.
Therefore, methods that clear lungs, relieve sore throat and remove obsta-
cles are usually adopted to eliminate pathological factors in the lung and
prevent it from transmitting to the spleen and kidneys, so that spleen and
kidney functions are not affected and metabolism of fluid remains normal. The key point is the thorough clearance of respiratory tract so the
pathological factors will be dispelled. In the recovery phase, deficiency in
spleen and kidney is usually obvious and should be the main focus of treatment. By regulating lung function while nourishing spleen and kidney, the
balance of the three organs is re-established in regulating fluid metabolism
and patients can soon recover.

Zhang Zhenyu suggested strengthening of the spleen as the treatment of diarrhea should be assisted by warming of the kidneys. This is

because spleen *yang* originates from kidney *yang*. When kidney *yang* is insufficient to warm the spleen, both organs will be deficient in *yang* and that results in diarrhea. When it becomes chronic, the kidneys will be affected, leading to decline of vital gate fire. Thus, Zhang often, in addition to nourishing spleen, gives Malaytea Scurfpea fruit, fortune's drynaria rhizome, Schisandra Chinensis, Alpinia Oxyphylla, Euryale Ferox, and lotus seed. This is also a reflection of "Treating Disease before Its Onset."

2.2.6 *Focus on recuperation, consolidate the therapeutic effect, control the factor triggering the disease, and prevent relapse*

Functions of body usually have not fully recovered shortly after diseases are cured. Therefore, relapse of the diseases is commonly seen if patients are not taken good care of. Zhang Zhongjing divides relapse according to causes into three categories: relapse due to diet, over-fatigue, and infections. Post-recovery care is emphasized by Zhang in order to avoid relapse.

Wang Mianzhi put asthma into one of the "diseases difficult to treat" as asthma has a long disease course and recurs easily. If only treated via resolving phlegm and invigorating kidney to improve ventilation, asthma can be controlled, but for a short period only. The reason for its relapse is normally the deficiency of spleen and lung due to its long disease course. Thus, invigoration of kidney to cut source for phlegm and reinforcement of *qi* and consolidation of superficies should be continued after patients having been relieved from asthma symptoms to prevent a relapse. Wang thinks the prevention and treatment of asthma requires attention to both symptoms and radicals. And treatment should include preventative measures for the long-term well-being of the patients.

Li Zhenhua has his own opinion in preventing relapse due to diet. In late stage of dampness-heat diseases, while heat is being gradually cleared, dampness cannot be rapidly removed. Provided that spleen *qi* is not fully recovered, stasis in circulation caused by spleen deficiency is often observed. Invigoration of spleen is then the priority to consolidate the therapeutic effect. Food light in taste and easy for digestion should be consumed rather than food that is raw, cold or heavy in taste. Doctors need to stress to patients that they should also have a controlled intake of food to avoid relapse due to improper diet.

Zhang Jingren suggests three tips in the health care of patients with gastroptosis. Firstly, patients are to improve fitness, especially fitness of abdominal muscles via sit-ups. In addition, patients are to maintain a stable and healthy mental condition. Last but not least, the diet needs to be adjusted to avoid over-intake of food or having habitual suppers. The trick is to have more meals a day but less food items, preferably those that are easily digested, in each meal.

As for chronic hepatitis, chronic nephritis and pyelonephritis, and some diabetes that have high rates of relapsing, Guo Ziguang suggests continuation of treatment necessary even after the parameters and markers in tests have normalized, to consolidate the therapeutic effect.

In summary, experience from the famous CM doctors is rich in thoughts and methods that imply the concept of "Treating Disease before Its Onset." It is our duty to discover, sort out, inherit and apply it, and make more use of it in the "Treating Disease before Its Onset Project."

References

Guo, S.Y., *et al.* (2008) *Collections of Li Zhenhua's Medical Case Records and Medical Monographs*, 1st edn. People's Medical Publishing House, Beijing.

Jiang, W., *et al.* (2002) The ideas of "Treating Disease before Its Onset." *J. Nanjing Univ. Tradit. Chin. Med.* **18**(4), 209–210.

Liu, B.C. (2002) *Liu Bichen's Clinical experience*, 1st edn. China Medical Scientific and Technology Press, Beijing.

Yan, D.X., *et al.* (2003) *Qi-Blood and Long Life*, 2nd edn. Shanghai Scientific and Technological Literature Publishing House, Shanghai.

Yin, Y.P., *et al.* (2003) *Chinese Modern Hundred Traditional Chinese Medicine Clinical Experts' Collection — Zha Yuming*, 1st edn. China Press of Traditional Chinese Medicine, Beijing.

Wang, X.P., *et al.* (2008) *Collections of Zhang Zhenyu's Medical Case Records, Medical Monographs and Medical Notes*, 1st edn. People's Medical Publishing House, Beijing.

Chapter 3

Theoretical Study of *"Preventive Treatment of Disease"* in Traditional Chinese Medicine

Lei Hong

Abstract

The theory of *"Preventive treatment of disease"* is from *Huangdi Neijing*. The connotation is extensive; such precautionary and forestall kind of prevention ideology has been a far-reaching influence to the later generation. It is an essential basic theory of Traditional Chinese Medicine. Accompanied with new conception of health, it enhances the practical implication of the *"Preventive treatment of disease"* theory and will become the most promising prospect for development in this century. *"Preventive treatment of disease"* should not be worded generally, rather, it mainly refers to taking advance measurement to prevent disease from occurring, developing, evolving, and recrudescing. *"Preventive treatment of disease"* covers 'prevention before diseases' and 'preventing disease from exacerbated'. 'Prevention before diseases' is again sub-divided into 'self-regulation during disease-free' and 'prevention on pathogenic factor' which is prevention before any disease occurs. 'Preventing disease from exacerbated' is also sub-divided into 'early treatment', which is to prevent the diseases prior its aggravation, to calm the non-pathogenic viscera in advance to prevent disease prior its development; and to prevent the disease from recrudesce and sequela.

Keywords: Preventive Treatment of Disease; Health Preservation; Sub-Healthy; Healthy Lifestyle.

3.1 Introduction

The ideology of *"Preventive treatment of disease"* is first mentioned in *Huangdi Neijing* during the period of Spring and Autumn Warring State. Though written a long time ago, nevertheless one have to admire this never fading scientific thoughts as reflected in many aspects as in medical treatment, governing a country, administrating a matter, and people management. Accordance to Suwen's *Great Theory on Spirit Regulation According to the Qi of the Four Seasons*, "The sages do not treat a formed disease but to treat only unformed disease, to govern an order situation and not when disordered. When a man falls sick and is treated with medicine, or governing a chaos situation, is an analogous to as digging a well when thirsty, or casting prick when engaged in battle, isn't it too late…?" Physician Sun Simiao in the Tang Dynasty categorized diseases into: "not yet ill," "about to ill," and "already ill," and pointed out that "eliminate the trouble before it arise, preventive treatment of a disease, treat the disease before troubles." Between lines implicates that "before troubles" is a views of health preservation to prevent diseases and recuperate in advance when about to fall ill. Such precautionary measure, forestalling kind of prevention ideology has a far-reaching impact to the later generation and it is an essential basic theory of Traditional Chinese Medicine. Accompanied by new health concepts, it enhances the practical implication of the theory — *"Preventive treatment of disease"* and will becoming the most promising development in this century. *"Preventive treatment of disease"* is to treat the disease prior to its occurrence, prior to its aggravation, prior to its development, prior to its recrudescence, and prior to its sequelae. Take precautionary measures to prevent the disease from occurring, developing, evolving, recrudescing, and developing into sequelae. It has a broad meaning, mainly in two aspects including 'prevention before disease' and 'preventing disease from exacerbating.' 'Prevention before diseases' is divided into 'self-regulation during disease-free' and 'prevention of pathogenic factor' as well as to changing the environment, eliminating the hidden pathogenic factor due to the environment, this is a prevention before the occurrence of the disease. 'Preventing disease from exacerbating' is divided into early treatment, to prevent the diseases prior its aggravation, to calm the non-pathogenic viscera in advance so as to prevent disease prior its development, and to prevent the disease from recrudesce and sequelae.

3.2 The Significances of *"Preventive Treatment of Disease"* in Health Preservation Science — Self-Regulation During Disease-Free

The *"Preventive treatment of disease"* in Health Preservation science focuses on self-regulation during disease-free. The main contents of the regulation are the regular pattern and rhythm of life. This is reflected in the respect of the body's own inherent law (functional regulation). Take the initiative to improve the adaptability with the natural world (orderliness regulation); as much as possible, avoid adverse interference in the course of life (habitué regulation); health preservation and self-cultivation are equally important, body and mind syncretism (psychology regulation), the purpose is to achieve a disease-free self-regulation health preservation. The key at this stage is to regulate steadily to avoid future misery.

3.2.1 *Functional regulation*

The TCM always deem the human body as an organism whole, an organic signify life, and life signify the movement of '*qi*' (*qi* movement). Holistic signify the uniformity coherence between the viscera and bowel functions. That is to say the '*qi*' of the human body viscera and bowel exist as in the concept of quantity distinguish as in 'existence,' 'non-existence,' 'strong,' 'weak,' 'great' and 'little.' At the same time whether there is a coordination between the '*qi*' of each viscera and bowel and they are interrelation. On this basis, there is a double meaning in TCM as regards to "reinforce the healthy *qi*": Firstly, the adequacy of the healthy *qi*: and secondly, is the coordination of human body *qi* movement. According to Suwen's *Method Discussion of the Reminding* chapter, "When the healthy *qi* store within, the pathogen is unable to interfere." The healthy *qi* is the vitality radiates from its own basic substance of the body organism. With the new conception of health, achieving the objective of "reinforce the healthy *qi*" begins with senescence health prevention and extends to strong physical health preservation, and youthful retaining health preservation. In other words, with the continued rising of living standards, the health care awareness of the society has increased. Health is not only to survive without diseases, it has to lead a better life, a quality life, and also to lead a beautiful and exciting life. This quality and excitement is no other than the healthy appearance and charm that radiates from the healthy *qi* of human body, and that is vitality.

Practically, it is whether the adequacy of healthy *qi* and the coordination of *qi* movement when implements onto health preservation science. Linshu's *Natural Life-span* pointed out that "five solid viscera, harmonious blood vessel, flexible muscles, compact skin, the orderly movement of nutrient-defense *qi*, smooth respiration, regular *qi* movement, well digestion of grains in six bowels, well-distributed body fluids, each as they often, therefore human could live longer." states that health preservation is about nourishing the healthy *qi* and nourishing the body functionality.

3.2.2 *Orderliness regulation*

In nature there are climate changes as in spring, summer, autumn, winter, as evolving into mankind and biosphere with the law of birth, growth, transformation, harvest and storage. Well-being cultivation during disease-free is premised on the respect of the law of nature and to seek the organism own regularity objectively. The TCM refer it as homologizing of heaven and man and is so-called the biological clock phenomenon. Linshu's *Generating and Meeting of Nutrient-Defense Qi* stated: "Men are endowed with *qi* from grains, when grains get into the stomach, it's transported to the lungs, five viscera and six bowels, each endowed with *qi*, the clear part act as the nutrient *qi*, the turbid part act as the defense *qi*, nutrient *qi* runs inside the vessels, defense *qi* runs outside the vessels, both running ceaselessly and meet once after fifty cycles. *Yin* and *yang* interlinked, like a ring without ending...." Linshu's *Carbuncle Gangrene* stated that: "therefore it travels because of breathing, travel in control, cycle with principle, concord with the heaven, without cease." It worth emphasizing that the cultivation of well-being during disease-free requires active regulation and not just passive adaptation. The ability of the human body in adapting to the nature is actually the balancing ability between the human body and the nature.

When implemented onto health preservation science it is the objective regularity of the coordination between the organism and nature. Health preservation is to cultivate the synchronization between man and nature.

3.2.3 *Habitué regulation*

Health preservation is not an overnight move, nor could a disease occur and develop within a short day; a disease breakout is always due to habitual unhealthy diet or irregular lifestyle over a long period of time. From birth, through growth to adulthood and aging, and finally death, the entire life process that takes several decades, which is relatively lengthy, just like a day. In order to maintain synchronization order between man and nature, it is difficult to achieve goal without persistent practice. A healthy lifestyle is the lifetime guarantee for health. Suwen's *Discussion of Heavenly Truth in Ancient Times* pointed out, "the one whom know the principle, follow with *yin* and *yang*, practice physical exercise appropriately, temperate in diets, leads a regular lifestyle, will not work against the routine, therefore, the spirits and body are complete and able to live to the utmost natural span of life. Whereas drinking wine as beverage, leads an abnormal lifestyle, having sexual intercourse when drunk, exhausting its essence by desires, dissipating its genuine *qi*, ignorance in sustaining fullness of *qi*, frequently tax on one's mind, hanker after a moment's pleasure, against the living pleasure, leads an irregular lives, therefore, decrepitude at the age of fifties."

In June 2006, the American Heart Association published an online updated version of diet and lifestyle recommendation. Unlike in the past, this round the AHA particularly emphasized on equally, changing of lifestyle and a reasonable diet; 80% of the cardiovascular disease can prevented through a healthy diet and lifestyle. It is impossible to actualize the standard of healthy lifestyles overnight, however, ultimately one can benefit from striving hard along this direction ceaselessly (Ma, 2006).

In all ages good rest and work habits, good diet habits, good exercise habits, good hygiene habits, good egests habits, good cuisine habits, and good recreation habits etc., are all important and it must be a persistence scientific lifestyle under the guidance of health awareness. To simplify a great truth, it is to do simple habits repeatedly; the purpose is to establish the order of the body function.

When implemented onto the health preservation science that is the cultivation of a persistence scientific lifestyle and cultivation of daily habits scientifically.

3.2.4 *Psychology regulation*

The human being is not only an organism it is also a social person with psychomotor activities. The human desires: happiness, anger, worry, thought, sorrow, fear, and shock, are the normal psychological reaction of human being in the social behavior. And the results of emotional change is interfering directly to the coordination function of the body *qi* movement, thus a well-controlled smooth body *qi* movement will avoid diseases whereas an uncontrolled disorder *qi* movement will develop diseases. Linshu's *The Master's Biography* pointed out, "Whether to govern people or self-governing, to govern a big or small matter, to govern a country or manage a household, it will not be able to govern it well if the approach is against one's will and this has to take the approach in an agreeable way. This is not just referring to the reverse and due circulations of the nutrient-defense *qi* within *yin* and *yang* meridians, it is like when treating the people, you have to listen to their wishes." "As for one's mental power is amiable then he will able to concentrate, the soul will not desultory, hatred and anger will not arise outrageously, therefore the five viscera are harmonious and will not harm by the pathogen *qi*."

The key issue of health preservation is that human emotions are in control. A normal person may behave abnormal psychologically. The occurrence of the disease, aggravation, transformation, and recrudesce etc. is resulted only under two conditions: as in sudden impetuosity, and long-term sustainment of unhealthy emotion. Therefore, other than the body discipline, in addition is the temperament cultivation, this is so-called nature-cultivation in addition to self-cultivation.

To implement onto the health preservation science is to learn to control unhealthy emotions, release unhealthy emotions with appropriate methods, and maintain peace of mind; this will ensured the coordination function of the human body. Control and regulate one's psychology, seek balances and steadiness in the dynamics society. As Suwen's *Discussion of Heavenly Truth in Ancient Times said*, the so-called "keep indifferent and nihility, reserve the truth of the heaven *qi*, the essence-sprit will defends within, ones will not suffer from diseases." More precisely, health preservation is all about nature cultivation.

3.3 The Significance of Preventive Treatment of Disease in Etiology Pathogenesis — Prevention on Pathogenic Factor

The TCM etiology pathogenesis believes that the occurrence of disease is the results of battles between the healthy and pathogenic *qi*. "Reinforce the healthy *qi*" is aimed at the results of human body healthy *qi* preservation. This is the prevention for senescence or self-regulation during disease-free;

the expulsion of the pathogenic *qi* is aiming at the results of the release of the disease pathogenic *qi* (aiming at pathogenic and environment factors). The meaning of *"Preventive treatment of disease"* in the aspect of etiology pathogens is mainly reflected with pertinence to defending against diseases. The key at this stage is to take preventive measures and expel the pathogenic *qi* without fail.

3.3.1 *Aiming at the pathogenic factor*

In the Ming Dynasty, China started its smallpox inoculation technique use for variola prevention — it is the world's pioneer in medical immunifaction. In 17th century, it not only had introduced the vaccination across the country but also spread it abroad. This had established the fundamental ideology of prevention for disease and extended the *Preventive treatment of disease* method in TCM. In Yuan Dynasty, Hua-Shou in his book *Book of Measles* proposed applying 消毒保婴丹 (*Xiaodu Baoying Dan*); 代天宣化丸 (*Dai Tian Xuanhua Wan*) during the measles epidemic season, which is clearly a record of using medicine as a preventive measure. In 1976 in the village of Shi-jia, Chinese medicinal was applied to prevent the spread of B meningitis. In the spring of 2003, Chinese medicinal played a pivotal role in controlling the spread of SARS across the country. These are the best examples of prevention for disease using the method of oral administration. Whether is in the past or future, preventing diseases from transmitling and developing into epidemics is an arduous task and the inoculation technique and oral medicinal cannot be ignored.

3.3.2 *Aiming at the environment*

Dating back in 2500 years ago, the knowledge of health and hygiene of China in the history of world medical had been very prominent. In personal hygiene, the people in the Xia and Shang Dynasty already have the habits of washing face, hands, legs and shower bath; people are more aware of shower in a regular basis during Chou Dynasty. As recorded in *The Book of Rites*, "In every five days, the younger will boil and prepare warm shower bath water for their parent, in every three days, the younger will boil and prepare warm water for their parent to wash their head. When their face gets dirty, wash

it with rice water, when their feet gets dirty wash it with warm water…"
"Gargle with salt water when the crowing is first heard in the morning…"
In the sanitation aspect people when through a long-term production, live-
lihood practices and gradually aware of the use of groundwater. According
to legend, there were already wells in the era of the Yellow Emperor and in
the era of Xia, the man named "Bo-Yi" is the inventor of wells. Among Yin
Ruins relics of the Shang era, underground drainage pipeline for discharging
excess water was found. In books such as Zhou Li's *Classic of Bureaucracy*,
Yi Li's *Classic of Etiquette* system, Shi Jing's *Classic of Poetry* etc., a great
deal of anti-pests and anti-rodent methods have been recorded. The Zhou
Dynasty are already known the measure and methods in sanitation and health
care such as the dredging of canals, discharge of water-logged, removal of
muck and slit in the wells during spring for new fresh water, anti-pest and
anti-rodent measures, and expulsion of mad dogs to prevent rabies. During
the period of Spring and Autumn Warring State, the people in China has the
habit to grid on "*lán-zhī*" (兰芷, a type of herbal) to avoid evil and epidemic prevention. At that time people fumigated herbs such as "*cang-zhu*"
(苍术, *Rhizoma Atractylodis*), "*xiong-huang*" (雄黄, Rabiagar), and "*ai-ye*"
(艾叶, Argy Wormwood leaf) etc. for epidemic prevention; fumigated "*pei-
lan*" (佩兰, Fortune Eupatorium herb) during the dragon boat festival, wore
bags containing herbals of "shi-chang-pu" (石菖蒲, Grassleaf Sweetfalg
Rhizome) and "*pei-lan*," and fumigated vinegar, etc. to prevent influenza.
This usage has become a custom that is practiced until now.

Presently the medicinal use for prophylaxis externally consist mainly of
fumigation medicinal, steaming medicinal, shower bath medicinal, grid-on
medicinal, pillow medicinal, compress medicinal, powder medicinal, etc.
The disease prevention measures not only have the inoculation technique
and oral medicinal, also the control and improvement conditions in the
environmental sanitation facility. The objective of the above is to make use
of all controllable measures to prevent disease invasion to human bodies.

3.4 The Significance of *Preventive Treatment of Disease* in Sub-Healthy

The so-called sub-healthy state is mostly without clinical symptoms
and signs, or there is conscious awareness of sensory symptoms but no
evidence of clinical examination. The message of the latency pathogenesis

trend is already exist and the body organism is at the state of structural and physiological function degradation with low quality of life and psychological imbalance condition. Generally, the sub-healthy state exhibits four modalities: (1) the state of fatigue and weakness that rules out the cause by disease; (2) the intermediate state between healthy and illness; (3) the state prior to disease, as in physical, psychological, social adaptability and moral being, health condition is less than perfect; and (4) the state where the age is incommensurate with the body structure and physiological function that is in declining condition, also known as 'third state.'

The so-called 'third-state' is refer to the body organism that has no significant disease but physiologically appear to be reduced in vitality, diminished in response, declined in adaptability, etc. It is mainly expressed as fatigue, weakness, dizziness, backache, easily infected with disease, etc. At this point the body shown clinical symptoms but without any laboratory examination indicator — this is at the stage of "about to fall ill." As Sun Simiao mentioned in *Qian jin yao fang*, "There are many people that suffers from physical discomfort as their energy and physical are not as good as before, they needs to know the method of health preservation and recuperation as soon as possible. If they are to endure the sickness without recuperate and thinking that it can be self-healed, then sooner it will develop into a pertinacious illness." As sub-healthy is a critical bidirectional state that lies between healthy and illness, it can moves towards the healthy state with reasonable well recuperation and maintenance, but will lead to disease due to quantitative change through lack of attention. This is a preparation stage of the disease change from a quantitative to qualitative. The body is always at a dynamic state that constantly changing, even a healthy person can be at the state of sub-healthy at a specific periods. The meaning of *"Preventive treatment of disease"* in the aspect of sub-healthy is mainly reflected in four patterns of manifestation: the application of treatment in accordance to syndromes, the application of recuperation in accordance to syndromes, the timely modulation, and the restoration of functionality of the body. This allows the body to returns to its equilibrium state timely and break away from the chain of "about to fall ill" and put an end to the disease occurrence.

The key at this stage rests with controllable and regulation of the health state.

3.5 The Significance of *Preventive Treatment of Disease* in Sub-Clinical

The so-called sub-clinical stage is when the disease had already occurred but the patient do not have any self-conscious symptoms. It is an exceptional stage where there is laboratory tests indications but with no clinical symptoms. This is difference from the sub-healthy as it is not at the stage of "not yet ill" or "about to fall ill" but it is at the stage of "already ill," this appertaining to the category of early treatment in *Preventive treatment of disease*. As early as in the Lingshu's *The Harmful Wind*, who pointed out, "There is some previous pathogen *qi* lingered within the body and yet to induce a disease. The *qi* and blood within the body becomes disorder as the results of feeling repulsion and admiration then the latent pathogen will wrestle with the emotional frustrations. The disease appears almost imperceptibly and is difficult to notice through looking and listening."

A research paper published in 2004 in *Circulation* indicated that in the years between 1984–1999, the mortality rate of the age group betweens 35–44 due to coronary heart disease in Beijing is increasing prominently; among the factors that causing the increasing mortality in coronary heart disease is cholesterol and that accounts for 77%. In addition, over the same period, a survey indicates that only 7% of the population aware of cholesterol abnormalities (Zhao, 2006). In other words, a vast majority of the cardiovascular and cerebrovascular incidents occurs within the "healthy" group. As we age, the phenomena of vascular aging is inevitable, we cannot reverse this phenomena but we can delay its progress. Atherosclerosis is the thickening and hardening of the arterial wall, a pathological process of gradual elasticity loss, and this change in the blood vessel wall structure is the basic cause of a cardiovascular incident.

The significances of the sub-clinical arteriosclerosis test is a comprehensive test carried out to evaluate the health of the blood vessel and to promptly prevent a vascular lesion; to prevent an incident from occuring when a vascular lesion had occurred; and to prevent a recurrence of a vascular event when patient had suffered from a vascular event. Hence, at the early stage, to be able to efficiently and accurately identify individuals that suffered from sub-clinical atherosclerosis from the public that appears healthy, this is the focal point of prevention strategy, and to take intervention in lifestyle at the early stage as risk factor control, the key is to prohibit and delay the development of atherosclerosis. Taking precautionary measures, and lowering the risk of severe cardio-cerebral vascular disease that may be in the future, also to serves the purpose of raising the standard of the national health care.

The meaning of *"Preventive treatment of disease"* in the sub-clinical aspect lies in timely prohibition of the disease from breaking out or aggravating, or to delay the disease from progression. The key of this stage is the foresight at early detection.

3.6 The Significance of *"Preventive Treatment of Disease"* in Clinical Prevention Science

When the disease occurred with clinical symptoms and changes in pathology with the laboratory evident, this is a typical stage of "already ill," this means that the body has emerged trauma and needs to carry out rehabilitation. However, diseases are classified into mild, severe, gradual, acute, likely to relapse or less recurrence, reversible or irreversible, uncomplicated or complicated. When the state of the disease is mild then it should prevented from aggravating; when the state of the disease is severe then it should prevented from deteriorating. The disease should be prevented from developing from acute to chronic due to procrastination treatment. Chronic disease should be prevented from complications and sequelae. A disease that is likely to relapse should be prevented from breaking out. A disease that is less recurrence should prevent an un-thorough treatment. Diseases that are reversible should be prevented from procrastination. Diseases that are reversible should be prevented from advancement. When the state of the disease is uncomplicated, then it should be prevented from getting into complication; when the state of the disease is complicated, then it should prevented from developing, etc. It does not mean that there would not be any "not-yet ill" preventive treatment after a disease had occurred. The meaning of "not-yet ill" is the forward-looking at every aspect of a disease. Zhang Zhongjing (one of the ancient medical scholars) mentioned in *Jin Gui Yao Lue* (first chapter, Ill Orderly of the Visceral and Meridians), "When liver disease surfaced, it is known that the disease will pass it on to the spleen, therefore need to fortify the spleen in advance." Ye Tian Shi mentioned in *Treatise on Warm Heat Disease*, "To first calm the unaffected area that has yet to suffers from pathogen," is the caution any prevention ideology puts forth about preventing illness from evolvement.

Although the clinical preventive measures are well recognized, the process of preventive treatment of disease may not be rigorous. For example, in the morbidity process of a chronic bronchitis to hypoxic pulmonary heart disease, in each chronic bronchitis attack the bronchial will become inflamed and the risk of pulmonary fibrosis will increase with each attack, and in TCM concept the blood stasis will also intensify with each attack. At this point in time it is important to have anti-inflammatory treatment, but one will also have to take consideration to activate blood (promote blood circulation and removing blood stasis) and resolve stasis. By the time after a few decades when the lips cyanosis symptoms finally emerged, it is indeed too late for the physician to think of activating blood and resolve stasis and for the patient to think of quitting smoking!

The meaning of "*Preventive treatment of disease*" in the clinical prevention study is about the concept of implementing treatment on different diseases, to manage it carefully in every step and to take prevention at each sector of the pathological change. The key elements at this stage depend very much on the doctor's standards and the patient's agreeability towards the treatment plan of the disease.

3.7 The Significance of *Preventive Treatment of Disease* in Clinical Recuperation Science

The so-called clinical recuperation is the process of preventing disability and sequela after the occurrence of a disease. From the analysis of three levels prevention objectives in clinical recuperate science: the first level of prevention is to prevent an occurrence of the disease and this is not classified under the category of clinical recuperation; the second level of prevention is to prevent the disease from aggravation, disability and dysfunction after it has occurred; and the third level of prevention is when the disease had induced disability and sequela, necessitating a recovery with time so as to avoid the recurrence of the primary disease. The crucial problem lies in after the disease had occurred, and successive preventive measures were carried out in every stage of the clinical treatment and recuperation. In TCM, the so-called disease recrudesce prevention is to prevent "recrudesce due to food", and "recrudesce due to fatigue" is a significant complement in clinical recuperation.

The meaning of *"Preventive treatment of disease"* in the clinical recuperation aspect lies in the prohibition of disability, sequela or recurrence in a timely manner. The key at this stage is the forward-looking in the sector of each pathological change.

In summary, the key of *"Preventive treatment of disease"* lies in prevention. This preventive awareness is the core and fundamental ideology of *"Preventive treatment of disease."* If we were to classify the disease stages "not yet ill," "about to fall ill," and "already ill," then with the health preservation as its objective, the stage of self-regulation during disease-free is the stage of "not yet ill." The stage of "about to fall ill" is refer to sub-healthy with clinical symptoms but without the laboratory tests indications and sub-clinical with laboratory tests indication but without clinical symptom; the disease at the stage of clinical treatment and recuperate treatment is at the stage of "already ill." *"Preventive treatment of disease"* covers all stages of "not-yet ill," "about-to ill," and "already ill" and the main ideology is prevention.

References

Ma, L.H. (2006) For health, to change our lifestyle — from the AHA recommendations. *China Medical Tribune* 29th June.

Zhao, S.P. (2006) Lipid-Regulation treatment and reversal of the coronary atherosclerosis. *China Medical Tribune* 6th July.

Chapter 4

Botanical Supplements for Aging

Harry H.S. Fong and Gail Mahady

Abstract

Aging is associated with numerous physiologic and psychosocial changes and with increased needs for medical care. Older adults are usually affected by two or more chronic diseases; are ill longer; have longer hospital stays; and hence, greater physical, mental and financial burdens. Complementary and alternative medicines (CAM), especially in the form of herbal medicines and botanical dietary supplements, are options that are being increasingly used by adults, including elderly consumers over 60 years of age, to treat or prevent a wide array of ailments such as chronic pain, arthritis, high cholesterol, insomnia, anxiety, Alzheimer disease, dementia, benign prostatic hyperplasia, and cardiovascular diseases. There are currently thousands of traditional medicines (TM) and other CAM herbal products available as such therapeutic agents worldwide. Yet, of the nearly 2000 herbal medicines listed in the Cochrane Controlled Trials Register as of June 2009, most of the clinical trials focus on a single plant herbal or phytomedicine. Hence, in this review, we will concentrate on single herb products that have been documented to have some clinical evidence of efficacy and/or safety for the treatment of diseases associated with aging. Space limitations, however, will not allow us to discuss every herbal product useful for this group of the population. In this review, the following herbs and their potential medical uses will be presented as examples of herbal medicine of potential relevance to the aging population. The examples presented are Boswellia (potentially useful for the management of arthritis, bronchial asthma, Crohn's disease, and ulcerative colitis), Echinacea (treatment and prevention of upper respiratory infections), Ginkgo (treatment and prevention of dementia), Ginseng (adaptogen for the maintenance and restoration of health, among other chronic conditions), Hawthorn (potential cardiovascular adjunct), Huperzia (Alzheimer's disease), Pygeum (Benign Prostatic Hyperplasia), and Saw Palmetto (Benign Prostatic Hyperplasia).

Keywords: Botanical Supplements; Aging; *Boswellia Echinacea*; Ginkgo;
Ginseng; Hawthorn; Huperzia; Pygeum; Saw Palmetto.

4.1 Introduction

With few exceptions, the segment of the pop over the age of 60 years is growing faster than any other age group in almost every country of the world. By
the year 2050, the world's population aged 60 years and over will have more
than tripled from 600 million in 2000 to 2 billion. Most of this increase will
be seen in developing countries, where the number of older people will rise
from 400 million in 2000 to 1.7 billion by 2050 (WHO, 2010).

By the year 2011, aging Americans will become an unprecedented segment of the U.S. population, as baby boomers (those born between 1946
and 1964) begin turning 65 years of age (Barnes and Bloom, 2008). In
general, most Americans are living longer lives due to significant improvements in healthcare, socioeconomic status, and health behaviours. In fact,
the fastest growing segment of the population is people over 85 years of
age. Thus, it is essential for older people to maintain good health in order
to remain independent, and life-long health promotion and disease prevention activities can prevent or delay the onset of non-communicable and
chronic diseases, such as heart disease, stroke and cancer (WHO, 2010).

However, currently older adults make up the segment of the population
that is the most diverse and at the highest risk for chronic diseases (NCHS,
2008). This demographic change has many implications for public health.
Aging is associated with numerous physiologic and psychosocial changes
and with increased needs for medical care. Thus, the trend of global population aging has led to a significant rise in the incidence of chronic diseases
and medical costs (NCHS, 2008; US-DHHS, 2000). Older adults are usually affected by more than two chronic diseases including cancer, heart
disease, hypertension, type 2 diabetes, stroke, dementia, metabolic disturbances and cirrhosis (Weekes *et al.*, 1999). Older adults are ill longer and
have longer hospital stays, and reportedly up to 55% of hospitalized older
adults are poorly nourished (Weekes *et al.*, 1999). Thus, there is a need for
new strategies for the prevention and treatment of chronic diseases.

Globally, there has been a resurgence in the interest of complementary and alternative medicines (CAM), especially in herbal medicines

and botanical dietary supplements (Kapoor *et al.*, 2009). Consumers in the United States are increasingly using complementary and alternative medicines (CAM) including botanicals to treat or prevent a wide array of ailments including the common cold, depression, and other non-life threatening medical conditions (Barnes *et al.*, 2004; Barnes and Bloom, 2008). In 2007, almost four out of ten adults had used CAM therapy in the past 12 months, with the most commonly used therapies being non-vitamin, non-mineral, natural products (17.7%) and deep breathing exercises (12.7%). American Indian or Alaska Native adults (50.3%) and white adults (43.1%) were more likely to use CAM than Asian adults (39.9%) or African American adults (25.5%) (Barnes and Bloom, 2008). Generally, persons who choose CAM approaches are seeking ways to improve their health and well-being (Austin *et al.*, 2000; Sebastian *et al.*, 2007; Wolosko *et al.*, 2002) or to relieve symptoms associated with chronic, even terminal, illnesses or the side effects of conventional treatments for them (Humpel *et al.*, 2006).

Between 30–41% of Americans aged 60 years or older have used at least one CAM modality, as compared with those younger than 60 years (Barnes *et al.*, 2004; Barnes and Bloom, 2008). Of this group of CAM users, 13–25% of people ages 60–85 used biologically-based CAM including dietary supplements (Barnes and Bloom, 2008). Interestingly, a large percentage of American adults are using CAM therapies to treat diseases associated with age, such as chronic pain, arthritis, high cholesterol, insomnia and anxiety (Barnes and Bloom, 2008). Along with non-botanical products such as fish oil (omega 3 or DHA), glucosamine and coenzyme Q, the list of commonly used botanicals include: ginseng, *Ginkgo biloba*, saw palmetto, garlic, and Echinacea (Barnes and Bloom, 2008). Other chronic conditions associated with aging include Alzheimer disease, dementia, benign prostatic hyperplasia, and cardiovascular disease.

Although there are currently thousands of traditional medicine (TM) and other CAM herbal products available as therapeutic agents worldwide. Yet, few of these products have been subjected to randomized clinical trials (RCTs) under ICH (International Conference on Harmonization good clinical practice (GCP) guidelines (www.ich.org) to determine their efficacy and/or safety. Of the nearly 2000 herbal medicine clinical studies listed on the Cochrane Controlled Trials Register as of June 2009, most of these concern single plant herbal or phytomedicine (www.mrw.interscience.wiley.com/cochrane). Hence, in this review, we will concentrate on single herb products that have been documented to have some evidence of efficacy and/or safety for the treatment of diseases associated with aging. Space limitation, however, will not allow us to discuss every herbal product useful for the aging. In this review, the following herbs, including *Boswellia Echinacea*, Ginkgo, Ginseng, Hawthorn, Huperzia, Pygeum, and Saw Palmetto, will be presented as examples of herbal medicine of potential relevance to the aging population.

4.2 Boswellia Resin

4.2.1 *Introduction*

Boswellia Gum Resin is the dried gum resin of *Boswellia serrata* Roxb. ex Colebr. (Burseraceae) and is also known as Gummi Boswellii, Gummi Guggul, and Frankincense, among other common names (Anon., 2000; Ayurvedic Pharm, 1999; WHO, 2009a). It has been employed as an anti inflammatory and anti-arthritic agent. Botanically, the source plant, a medium to large sized deciduous tree up to 18 m in height and 2.4 m in girth with imparipinnate leaves, is also known by its synonyms, *Boswellia glabra* Roxb., *B. thurifera* (Colebr.) Roxb. (Anon., 2000; List and Horhamme, 1975). The plant is native to India (Anon., 2000; Nadkarni, 1954; Kapoor, 1990). The plant part of interest is the gum-resin, which solidifi es slowly with time. It is reddish brown, greenish yellow, or dull yellow to orange in colour. It occurs in small, ovoid, fragrant tears. Sometimes the tears form agglomerated masses up to 5 cm long and 2 cm thick. Fracture is brittle, fractured surface is waxy and translucent. It burns readily and emanates an agreeable characteristic balsamic resinous odor. (Anon, 2000; Ayurvedic Pharm, 1999).

4.2.2 *Chemistry*

Chemically, the dried gum-resin contains 5–9% essential oil with major constituents being α-thujene (50–61%), sabinene (5%), α-pinene (8%) and

α-phellandrene (2%). Major triterpene constituents of biological interest are members of the boswellic acids (more than 12) including 11-keto-α-boswellic acid, 3-α-acetyl-11-keto-β-boswellic acid, α-boswellic acid, β-boswellic acid, 3-acetyl-β-boswellic acid, and 3-acetyl β-boswellic acid, (List and and Horhamme, 1975; Girgune and Garg, 1979; Verghese *et al.*, 1987; Wichtl, 2002).

4.2.3 *Clinical pharmacology*

Products containing *Boswellia serrata* are used for the management of arthritis, bronchial asthma, Crohn's disease and ulcerative colitis (Gerhardt *et al.*, 2001; Gupta *et al.*, 1997; 1998; 2001; Kimmatkar *et al.*, 2003; Nadkarni *et al.*, 1954; WHO, 2009a).

4.2.4 *Rheumatoid arthritis*

A double-blind pilot study, involving 37 patients with rheumatoid arthritis (RA), assessed the effects of the crude drug on the symptoms of swelling and pain of RA, and self-medication with non-steroidal anti- infl ammatory drugs (NSAID) (Sander *et al.*, 1998). Patients were treated with 3.6 g of the resin or placebo for 12 weeks. Outcomes measures included Ritchies index for swelling and pain, and the NSAID dose taken daily by the patients. There were no subjective, clinical or laboratory parameters showing significant reduction in pain and swelling changes from baseline to 12 weeks of treatment (Sander *et al.*, 1998).

A randomized double blind placebo controlled crossover study assessed the efficacy, and safety of a *B. serrata* extract (BSE) in 30 patients with osteoarthritis of knee, 15 subjects received the active BSE or placebo for eight weeks. After the first treatment, a washout period of was permitted and then the groups were crossed over to receive the opposite intervention for eight weeks. All patients receiving BSE treatment reported a reduction in knee pain, increased knee flexion and walking distance. The frequency of swelling in the knee joint was decreased, but radiologically there was no change. The observed differences between drug treatment and placebo were statistically signifi cant ($p < 0.05$). BSE was well tolerated by the subjects except for minor gastrointestinal adverse events. (Kimmatkar *et al.*, 2003).

4.2.5 *Bronchial asthma*

A double-blind, placebo-controlled study involving 40 patients with bronchial asthma assessed the effects of a *B. serrata* extract (BSE) for symptomatic treatment. The patients were treated with 300 mg of BSE three times daily for a period of six weeks. After treatment, 70% of patients showed improvement of disease as evident by disappearance of physical symptoms and signs such as dyspnoea, bronchial asthma, number of attacks, as well as a decrease in eosinophilic count and ESR. In the control group, patients treated with lactose 300 mg three times daily for six weeks, 27% of patients receiving the placebo also showed improvement. The data show a role for the crude drug in the treatment of bronchial asthma (Gupta *et al.*, 1998).

4.2.6 *Crohn's disease*

A randomized, double-blind, controlled, parallel group comparison clinical trial involving 102 patients assessed the effects of the crude drug for the treatment of Crohn's disease (Gerhardt *et al.*, 2001). The positive control arm was treated with mesalazine. The primary outcome measure was the change of the Crohn's Disease Activity Index (CDAI) between the time of enrolment and end of therapy. The CDAI was reduced by 90% after treatment with the crude drug and reduced by 53% with mesalazine. However, the difference between both treatments was not statistically significant. Thus, the study concluded that an extract of the crude drug was as effective as mesalazine for the treatment of Crohn's disease (Gerhardt *et al.*, 2001).

4.2.7 *Ulcerative colitis*

The effect of *B. serrata* resin in patients suffering from ulcerative colitis grades II and III was assessed in a comparison control study (Gupta *et al.*, 1997). Patients were treated with *B. serrata* resin preparation (350 mg three times daily for six weeks), and the effects on stool properties, histolopathology and scan microscopy of rectal biopsies, blood parameters including hemogloblin, serum iron, calcium, phosphorus, proteins, total leukocytes and eosinophils were measured. Patients receiving sulfasalazine (1 g three times daily) served as controls. At the end of the treatment period, all parameters tested improved in patients treated with *B. serrata* resin, the results being similar compared to controls: 82% out of treated patients went into remission; in the case of sulfasalazine, the remission rate was 75% (Gupta *et al.*, 1997). No statistical analysis of this study was performed.

A controlled clinical trial assessed the efficacy of the crude drug in patients with chronic colitis characterized by vague lower abdominal pain, bleeding per rectum with diarrhea and palpable tender descending and sigmoid colon. Thirty patients, 17 males and 13 females in the age range of 18 to 48 years with chronic colitis, were included in the study. Twenty patients were given a preparation of the *B. serrata* resin, at a dose of 300 mg three times daily for six weeks and ten patients were given sulfasalazine, at a dose of 1 g three times daily for six weeks and served as controls. Out of 20 patients treated with *B. serrata* resin, 18 patients showed an improvement in one or more of the parameters: stool properties, histopathology as well as scanning electron microscopy, besides hemoglobin, serum iron, calcium, phosphorus, proteins, total leukocytes and eosinophils. Out of 20 patients treated with *B. serrata* resin, 14 went into remission while in the case of sulfasalazine, the remission rate was four out of ten (Gupta *et al.*, 2001).

A systematic review of seven (out of 47) randomized clinical trials was recently published (Ernst, 2008). All studies were published between 1998 and 2008. The methodological quality of the trials was variable but three trials reached the maximum of 5 on the Jadad scale (Ernst, 2008). Five of the trials were placebo controlled and two were comparisons against active treatments. All studies used *B. serrata* extracts, administered orally. The review concluded that *Boswellia* extracts showed some promise in treating asthma, rheumatoid arthritis, Crohn's disease, knee osteoarthritis, and collagenous colitis. However, all trials had flaws, of which the most common limitations were small sample size and incomplete reporting of data. The largest study included 102 patients. Adverse effects of *B. serrata* were minor and were judged as not causally related to the treatment and not markedly different from those noted in the placebo groups (Table 4.1). Diarrhea and abdominal pain were the most common adverse events (Ernst, 2008; Singh *et al.*, 1996).

4.3 *Echinacea*

4.3.1 Introduction

Commercial *Echinacea* extracts are manufactured primarily from three *Echinacea* species: *Echinacea purpurea* (herb, roots, or seeds), *E. angustifolia* (roots), and *E. pallida* (roots). These products are used by oral administration for the prophylaxis and treatment of the common cold, bronchitis, influenza, and bacterial and viral infections of the respiratory tract, all of which the elderly are vulnerable to. The genus *Echinacea* is native to North America. *E. angustifolia* and *E. pallida* were considered to be varieties of the same species at one time. A considerable amount of *E. angustifolia* cultivated in Europe prior to the mid-1980s was indeed *E. pallida*. *Echinacea* species are hardy, herbaceous perennials with either simple or branched stems. The branches of *E. angustifolia* and *E. pallida* are simple and rarely branched, attaining heights of 10–50 and 40–90 cm, respectively, whereas, the stems of *E. purpurea* are erect, stout and branched, 60–180 cm in height (WHO, 1999a).

4.3.2 *Chemistry*

Chemically, at least five groups of chemical constituents have been identified in *Echinacea* species, and all are reported to contribute biologically, to the herbs' overall effectiveness. These five groups consist of the alkamides, polyalkenes, polyalkynes, caffeic acid derivatives, and polysaccharides. The volatile oil contains, among other compounds, borneol, bornyl acetate, pentadeca-8(Z)-en-2-one, germacrene D, caryophyllene and caryophyllene epoxide. In the alkamide group, isobutylamides of C11–C16 straight chain fatty acids with olefinic and/or acetylenic bonds are found in the aerial parts of all three species, with the isomeric dodeca-2E,4E,8Z,10E/Z-tetraenoic acid isobutylamides as the major active compounds of this group. More than 20 similar alkamides are found in the roots, with the highest concentration being in *E. angustifolia,* followed by *E. purpurea,* with the lowest concentration found in *E. pallida*. The main alkamide of the roots is a mixture of isomeric dodeca-2,4,8,10-tetraenoic acid isobutylamides. The caffeic acid ester derivative cichoric acid is the major active compound of this class found in the aerial parts, with the highest concentration being found in *E. purpurea* (1.2–3.1%), followed by *E. pallida,* with *E. angustifolia* (traces) a distant third. Echinacoside, on the other hand, is the major caffeic acid derivative in *E. angustifolia* (0.1–1.0%), but is found only in trace amounts in *E. pallida* and is totally absent from *E. purpurea.* Verbascoside (acetoside) has been reported in *E. angustifolia* and *E. pallida,* while cichoric acid methyl ester is also found in *E. purpurea.* The polysaccharides are immunostimulant constituents, two types from *E. purpurea*: a heteroxylan with an average molecular weight of 35 kD and an arabinorhamnogalactan of average molecular weight of 0.45 kD. Trace amounts of pyrrolizidine alkaloids (tussilagine [0.006%] and isotussilagine) have also been reported. While some pyrrolizidine alkaloids are hepatotoxic, the *Echinacea* pyrrolizidine alkaloids, due to their lack of a 1,2-unsaturated necine ring, are not. (Mahady *et al.,* 2001; WHO, 1999a).

4.3.3 *Clinical pharmacology*

Treatment and prevention of upper respiratory tract infections

Reviews of the clinical literature for *Echinacea* prior to 2001 have been published and are beyond the scope of this review (Mahady *et al.,* 2001b; WHO, 1999a). A more recent Cochrane review (Linde *et al.,* 2006) of sixteen clinical trials compared an *Echinacea* preparation and a control group (13 with placebo, two with no treatment, one with another herbal preparation). All trials except one were described as double-blind. Three clinical trials investigated *Echinacea* for the prevention of colds and 19 comparisons tested *Echinacea* products for the treatment of colds. The outcomes assessed in the prevention trials were: numbers of individuals with one or more colds, and severity and duration of colds; and in treatment trials: total symptom scores, nasal symptoms, and the duration of colds. A variety of different *Echinacea* preparations were used in the clinical trials. None of the three comparisons in the prevention trials showed an effect over the placebo. When comparing an *Echinacea* preparation with placebo as treatment, there is some evidence that preparations based on the aerial parts of *Echinacea purpurea* may be effective for the early treatment of colds in adults, however, and preventive the results are not fully consistent.

Beneficial and preventative effects of other *Echinacea* preparations might exist but have not been shown in independently replicated, rigorous randomized trials (Linde *et al.*, 2006).

A meta-analysis evaluated the effect of *Echinacea* products on the incidence and duration of the common cold (Shah *et al.*, 2007). Fourteen clinical studies were included in the meta-analysis. Incidence ($n = 1356$) of the common cold was reported as an odds ratio (OR) with 95% CI, and duration ($n = 1630$) of the common cold was reported as the weighted mean difference (WMD) with 95% CI. *Echinacea* treatment decreased the odds of developing the common cold by 58% (OR 0.42; 95% CI 0.25–0.71; Q statistic $p < 0.001$) and the duration of a cold by 1.4 days (WMD −1.44, −2.24 to −0.64; $p = 0.01$). Similarly, significant reductions were observed during subgroup analyses were limited to Echinaguard/Echinacin use, concomitant supplement use, method of cold exposure, Jadad scores less than three, or use of a fixed-effects model. Published evidence supports *Echinacea's* benefit in decreasing the incidence and duration of the common cold (Shah *et al.*, 2007).

The clinical data supporting the use of products containing *Echinacea* are confl icting (Woelkart *et al.*, 2008). There is an indication that preparations from the aerial parts and roots of *Echinacea purpurea* may be effective. However, more studies with precisely standardized products (pressed juices and tinctures), using rigorous clinical standards are necessary. So far in preventative trials, only a trend in reducing the development and severity of colds could be demonstrated, but this was not statistically significant. Preparations containing *Echinacea angustifolia* and *E. pallida* roots need further controlled clinical trials, in order to provide a better evidence for clinical effi cacy (Woelkart *et al.*, 2008).

4.4 Ginkgo

4.4.1 *Introduction*

Ginkgo is a monotypic dioecious plant that is the only living representative of the Ginkgoales. The seed kernel has been used as a culinary and medicine in China over the millennium (Keys, 1976; Pharmacopoeia PRC, 1992), while the leaf has been used as a phytomedicine and dietary supplement in more recent times in Western countries purportedly useful as a memory enhancer, particularly in the elderly population. The ginkgo plant has a number of vernacular names, including maidenhair tree, temple balm, *yin guo*, and *yinhsing* (DeFeudis, 1991; Hansel *et al.*, 1994; Huh and Staba, 1992). The ginkgo tree reaches a height of 35 m and a diameter of 3–4 m; has a grey bark; and fan-like green leaves that are deciduous, alternate, lengthily petiolate, base wedge-shaped, 6–9 cm broad (sometimes up to 15–20 cm). The dried leaves are green, grey-yellow, brown or blackish (Huh and Staba, 1992). Ginkgo is native to China, but is also grown as an ornamental shade tree in Australia, South-East Asia, Europe, Japan, and the United States of America (DeFeudis, 1991; Hansel *et al.*, 1994; Keys, 1976). It is commercially cultivated in France and the United States of America (Hansel *et al.*, 1994).

4.4.2 *Chemistry*

Chemically, the major constituents are flavonoids based on the fl avonols kaempferol and quercetin containing one, two or three glycosides and coumaric acid esters. Most importantly, the leaves contain as characteristics constituents, the unique diterpene lactones, ginkgolides A, B, C, J and M, as well as the sesquiterpene lactone bilobalide (Sticher, 1993; 1994).

4.4.3 *Clinical pharmacology*

4.4.3.1 *Treatment of dementia*

Extracts of the leaves of *Ginkgo biloba* (GBE), have long been used in medicine for cardiovascular diseases, as well as for the treatment of dementia (Birks *et al.*, 2009; Mahady *et al.*, 2001; WHO, 1999b). GBE is currently used for the management of age-associated memory impairment, which includes symptoms such as concentration problems, confusion, depression, anxiety, dizziness, tinnitus and headache (Birks *et al.*, 2009). The mechanisms of action include antioxidant and anti-infl ammatory effects, increasing blood supply by dilating blood vessels, reducing blood viscosity, modification of neurotransmitter systems (Birks *et al.*, 2009).

The most recent Cochrane review (Birks *et al.*, 2009) of the safety and efficacy of ginkgo for treatment of dementia analyzed 36 randomized, double-blind studies, in which GBE at any dose given over a variety of time periods, were compared with placebo for their effects on people with acquired cognitive impairment, including dementia, of any degree of severity. Most of the studies were small and less than three months in duration. Nine trials were of six months duration (2016 patients). These longer trials were of adequate size, and conducted with reasonably sound methodology. Most trials tested the same GBE, EGb 761, at different doses. The results of the systematic review showed that data from the more recent trials had inconsistent outcomes for cognition, activities of daily living, mood, and depression. Three studies found no difference between EGb 761 and placebo, and one study found a very large treatment effect in favor of EGb 761. Adverse event reporting for both the placebo and EGb 761 groups were similar. The review concluded that while EGb 761 appears to be safe, however the data demonstrating the efficacy of Gingko extracts for dementia or cognitive impairment is still inconsistent (Birks *et al.*, 2009)

Another review of the clinical trials assessed the efficacy of EGb 761 in the treatment of dementia (Alzheimer's disease and vascular dementia). Ten randomized, controlled, double-blind clinical trials, including the four large more recent studies, were reviewed. Three of the four large trials demonstrated that EGb 761 was significantly superior to placebo with respect to cognitive performance, and one or more further (global, functional or behavioural) outcomes demonstrating the clinical relevance of the findings. The results from the six smaller trials supported that of the larger trials. One trial was inconclusive, but of questionable external validity due to uncommonly rigorous patient selection. Subgroup analyses of this study together with the findings from the most recent clinical trial suggest that EGb 761 may be most beneficial to patients with neuropsychiatric symptoms. One exploratory trial comparing EGb 761 and donepezil (cholinesterase inhibitors) showed no statistically significant or clinically relevant differences. The review concluded that GBE was as effective as low doses of donepezil (Kasper *et al.*, 2009).

4.4.3.2 *Prevention of dementia*

A multicenter randomized, double-blind, placebo-controlled clinical trial was conducted to determine effectiveness of GBE vs placebo in reducing the incidence of all-cause dementia and Alzheimer disease (AD) in elderly individuals with normal cognition and those with mild cognitive impairment (MCI) (DeKosky *et al.*, 2008). At the study entry, 3069 community volunteers, aged 75 years or older, with normal cognition (*n* = 2587) or MCI (*n* = 482) were assessed every six months for incident dementia, and median follow-up was 6.1 years. The patients were treated with a twice-daily dose of 120 mg extract of GBE (*n* = 1545) or placebo (*n* = 1524). The main outcome measured was the incidence of dementia and AD as determined by expert panel consensus. The results of this trial showed that 523 individuals developed dementia (246 receiving placebo and 277 receiving GBE) with 92% of the dementia cases classified as possible or probable AD, or AD with evidence of vascular disease of the brain. The adverse effect profiles were similar for both groups. In this study, GBE at a dose of 120 mg twice a day was not effective in reducing either the overall incidence rate of dementia or AD incidence in elderly individuals with normal cognition or those with MCI (DeKosky *et al.*, 2008).

4.5 Ginseng

4.5.1 *Introduction*

Ginseng is the common name used in recent years for members of a taxonomically diverse group of at least 30 different species (Mahady *et al.*, 2001a). However, "ginseng" is derived from the Chinese word "*jen-shen*", which was roughly translated as "man-root" as the shape of the roots can resemble the human body (Hu, 1976; Awang, 2003). This particular plant was botanically identified as being a species of *Panax*, which is derived from the Greek word "panacea" (cure-all), although the concept that ginseng is a general "cure-all" is not correct (Hu, 1976; Sonnenborn and Proppert, 1991). Botanically, only products of *Panax* species should be referred to as "ginseng" (Awang, 2003). Of the nine species of *Panax*, the two most commercially important are *P. ginseng* and *P. quinquefolius*. Hence, the discussions in this chapter will be limited to these two species.

4.5.2 *Panax ginseng*

The primary commercial species, known scientifi cally as *Panax ginseng* C.A. Meyer (Araliaceae), originally named *Panax schinseng* Nees (Awang, 2003; WHO, 1999c), is commonly referred to as Korean,

Oriental or Asian ginseng. In China, the root or rhizome (underground stem) and the leaves of *P. ginseng* have been used medically (Hu, 1976). However, the root is the most prominent part and dominates the commercial market. The plant is a slow-growing perennial herb, with characteristic brqaanched-roots extending from the midddle of the main root in the form of a human fi gure. The main root is fusiform or cylindrical, 2.5–20 cm in length by 0.5–3.0 cm in width, which is usually not harvested until the 5th or 6th year of growth, when the biologically active ginsenosides are at the highest concentration (Hu, 1976; WHO, 1999c). Commercially, two major forms of *P. ginseng* root, white and red, are produced as a result of processing. White ginseng is the dried, bleached (sulfur dioxide) root of *P. ginseng*, sometimes peeled to remove the outer coating (skin) of the root. Red ginseng, on the other hand, is prepared by steaming the root followed by air-drying (Hu, 1976; Shibata *et al.*, 1985). The plant is indigenous to the mountain regions of Korea, Japan, China (Manchuria), and Russia (eastern Siberia) (Hu 1976). However, most commercial ginseng is now cultivated, as wild *P. ginseng* is now an endangered and protected species in both Russia and China (Carlson, 1986), with commercial products being prepared from cultivated ginseng, imported from China, Japan, Korea and Russia (Hu, 1976).

4.5.3 *Panax quinquefolius*

The second most important commercial species is the dried roots of *Panax quinquefolius* L. (Araliaceae), which has the synonyms of *Aralia quinquefolia* Dec. & Planch., *Ginseng quinquefolium* Wool, *Panax americanum* Raf. (WHO, 2009), is commonly referred to as American ginseng. This herb is highly prized in China, with most of the roots produced in North America being exported to the Orient via the port of Hong Kong since the 1970s, with a shipment of 55 tons being recorded as being sailed from Boston (USA) to China in 1773 (Tyler *et al.*,1981). The plant is a perennial herb, up to more than 1 m high. The root is fusiform, cylindrical or conical, 1–12 cm, sometimes up to 20 cm in length, and up to 2.5 cm in diameter at the crown, with one or or stem scars. Externally pale yellow to golden, exhibiting transverse-striations and linear-lenticels, and showing fine and dense longitudinal-wrinkles, and rootlet scars. *P. quinquefolius* is native to the United States and Canada, but is an endangered species. It is presently cultivated with the major production areas being Wisconsin (USA), Ontario (Canada), British Columbia (Canada) and northern China. The root is collected in the autumn, washed clean, and dried in the sun or at a low temperature (HKCMMS, 2009).

4.5.4 *Chemistry*

The main chemical constituents of *Panax ginseng* are the triterpene saponins, known as the ginsenosides. More than 30 are based on the dammarane structure, with one, ginsenoside Ro, being an oleanolic acid derivative (WHO, 1999c; Shibata *et al.*, 1985; Cui *et al.*, 1995; Sprecher, 1987). The ginsenosides are derivatives of either protopanaxadiol or protopanaxatriol. Members of the former group include the ginsenosides Ra-1,-2,-3; ginsenosides Rb–1, -2, -3; ginsenosides Rc, Rc-2; ginsenosides Rd, Rd-2; ginsenoside Rh-2; 20(S)-ginsenoside Rg-3; malonyl-ginsenosides Rb-1; malonyl-ginsenoside Rb-2; malonyl-ginsenosides Rc; and malonyl-ginsenoside Rd. Examples of protopanaxatriol saponins are: ginsenosides Re, -2, -3; ginsenoside Rf; 20-gluco-ginsenoside Rf; ginsenosides Rg-1, -2; 20(R)-ginsenoside Rg-2; 20(R)-ginsenoside Rh-1; and ginsenoside Rh-1 (WHO, 1999c). The most important constituents are the ginsenosides Rb-1, -2, Rc, Rd, Rf, Rg-1, and Rg-2 (WHO, 1999c). As in the case of *P. ginseng*, the ginsenosides of *P. quinquefolius* are derivatives of protopanaxadiol or protopanaxatriol, with the majority of these compounds (e.g. ginsenosides Rb1, Rb2, Rc, Rd, Re, Rg1, Ro) being common to both species. However, there are quantitative and qualitative differences. The total ginsenoside content of *P. quinquefolius* is higher than that of *P. ginseng*. At the same time, ginsenosides Rf and Rg2 do not occur in *P. quinquefolius*. On the other hand, 24(R)-pseudoginsenoside F11 is found in *P. quinquefolius*, but not in *P. ginseng*. In cultivated *P. quinquefolius*, however, the most dominant ginsenosides are malonyl (m)-Rbl, Rb1, and Re with the percentages of m-Rb1 and Rb1 being almost identical (Rg1 levels and total ginsenosides are much higher in wild than in cultivated *P. quinquefolius*) (Awang, 2000). Furthermore, the combined amounts of Rbl and m-Rb1 in often exceed one-half of the total ginsenoside content with the total malonyl ginsenoside (m-Rb1, m-Rb2, m-Rc, and m-Rd) content being approximately 40% (Awang, 2000; WHO, 2009b). In a study of wild American ginseng, total ginsenosides range from 1–16%, with the majority being 4–5% (Assinewe *et al.*, 2003). Polysaccharides of biological significance include quinquefolans A,B, and C (Oshima *et al.*, 1987).

4.5.5 *Panax ginseng: clinical pharmacology*

The traditional Chinese medical use of *Panax ginseng* is for the treatment of older patients with chronic illnesses, and it is especially given during periods of convalescence, to restore the person to a normal state of good health (Hu, 1976; Mahady *et al.*, 2001a). According to the World Health Organization, *Panax ginseng* is administered as a tonic or immune stimulant for enhancement of mental and physical capacity during fatigue, chronic illness, and convalescence (WHO, 1999c; Mahady *et al.*, 2001).

4.5.6 *Alzheimer disease*

One of the signifi cant effects of ginseng in the elderly is its positive effect on cognition. Recent experimental evidence indicates that ginseng administration has protective and trophic effects on memory in cases of Alzheimer disease (AD) (Lee *et al.*, 2008). One clinical trial investigated the effi cacy of *Panax ginseng* on cognitive performance in AD patients in an open-label study (Lee *et al.*, 2008). Consecutive AD patients were randomly assigned to the ginseng ($n = 58$) or the control group ($n = 39$), and the ginseng group was treated with powdered *Panax ginseng* root (4.5 g/d) for 12 weeks. Cognitive performance was monitored using the mini-mental state examination (MMSE) and Alzheimer disease assessment scale (ADAS) at the baseline and end of the trial. At baseline the MMSE and ADAS scales showed no difference between the groups. After ginseng treatment, the cognitive subscale of ADAS and the MMSE score showed improvements at 12 weeks ($p = 0.029$ and $p = 0.009$ vs. baseline, respectively). After discontinuing ginseng, the improved ADAS and MMSE scores declined to baseline. The results of this study suggest that *Panax ginseng* is clinically effective for improving cognitive performance of AD patients (Lee *et al.*, 2008).

4.5.7 *Dementia*

In a second study, the efficacy of Korean red ginseng (KRG; *Panax ginseng*) was investigated as an adjuvant therapy to conventional anti- dementia medications in patients with Alzheimer's disease (Heo *et al.*, 2008). A 12-week randomized study, involving 61 patients (24 males and 37 females) with Alzheimer's disease were randomly assigned to one of the following treatment groups: low-dose KRG (4.5 g/day, n = 15), high-dose KRG (9 g/day, n = 15) or control (n = 31). The Alzheimer's Disease Assessment Scale (ADAS), Korean version of the Mini-Mental Status Examination (K-MMSE) and Clinical Dementia Rating (CDR) scale were used to assess changes in cognitive and functional performance at the end of the 12-week study period. The results of this study showed that patients in the high-dose KRG group showed significant improvement on the ADAS and CDR after 12 weeks as compared with those in the control group (p = 0.032 and 0.006 respectively). The KRG treatment groups also showed improvement from baseline MMSE when compared with the control group (1.42 vs. −0.48), but this improvement was not statistically signifi cant. KRG showed good efficacy for the treatment of Alzheimer's disease; however, further studies with larger samples of patients and a longer effi cacy trial should be conducted to confirm the efficacy of KRG (Heo *et al.*, 2008).

4.5.8 *Reduced mortality*

One recent study investigated the association between *Panax ginseng* intake and mortality among the elderly members of the Korean population (Yi *et al.*, 2009). In the study, 6282 subjects who were 55 years of age or older in March 1985 until December 31, 2003, were followed over 18.8 years in a progressive cohort study. The Cox proportional hazard regression model was used to evaluate effects of ginseng intake on mortality. After adjusting for age, education, occupation, drinking, smoking, self-reported chronic disease, body mass index, and blood pressure, all-cause mortality for male ginseng users was significantly lower than that for male non-users (Hazard ratio [HR] = 0.90; 95% confidence interval [CI], 0.81–0.99). However, such an association was not observed in women (HR = 1.03; 95% CI, 0.94–1.13). Cancer-specific mortality was lower in female ginseng users than female non-users after adjustment of relevant covariates (HR = 0.80; 95% CI, 0.60–1.08). Compared to non-users, the HR for cancer-specific mortality in women was 0.84 in infrequent users (95% CI, 0.62–1.15) and 0.61 in frequent users (95% CI, 0.32–1.14) (p for trend, 0.09), which is not statistically signifi cant. The cancer specific mortality was not associated with ginseng intake in male subjects (HR = 0.95; 95% CI, 0.76–1.20). Mortality caused by cardiovascular diseases was not related to ginseng intake in both men and women (Yi *et al.*, 2009).

4.5.9 *Erectile dysfunction*

A systematic review evaluated the current evidence for the effectiveness of red ginseng (*Panax ginseng*) for treatment of erectile dysfunction (Kim *et al.*, 2008). All randomized clinical studies (RCT) of red ginseng as a treatment of erectile dysfunction were considered for inclusion. Methodological quality was assessed using the Jadad score, and seven RCTs met all the inclusion criteria, however their methodological quality was low on average. Six of the included RCTs compared the therapeutic efficacy of red ginseng with placebo. The meta-analysis of these data showed a significant effect (n = 349, risk ratio, 2.40; 95% CI of 1.65, 3.51, p < 0.00001, heterogeneity: tau(2) = 0.05, chi(2) = 6.42, p = 0.27, I(2) = 22%). Subgroup analyses also showed beneficial effects of red ginseng in psychogenic erectile dysfunction (n = 135, risk ratio, 2.05; 95% CI of 1.33, 3.16, p = 0.001, heterogeneity: chi(2) = 0.08, p = 0.96, I(2) = 0%). Collectively these RCTs provide suggestive evidence for the effectiveness of red ginseng in the treatment of erectile dysfunction. However, the total number of RCTs included in the analysis, the total sample size and the methodological quality of the primary studies were low (Kim *et al.*, 2008).

A double-blind, placebo-controlled study was conducted with 143 patients experiencing ED. Over the course of eight weeks, one group took 1000 mg of a *Panax ginseng* extract (TMGE) twice a day, and the other group took 1000 mg of placebo twice a day. The effects of the TMGE and the placebo were analyzed using the Korean version of the International Index of Erectile Function (IIEF) questionnaire. A total of 86 patients completed eight weeks of treatment. The scores on the five domains of the IIEF after medication were significantly higher than the baseline scores in the group treated with TMGE ($p < 0.05$), whereas no signifi cant improvement was observed in the placebo group ($p > 0.05$). Erectile function and overall satisfaction scores after medication were significantly higher in the TMGE group than in the placebo group ($p < 0.05$). Erectile function of patients in the TMGE-treated group significantly improved, suggesting that TMGE could be utilized for improving erectile function in male patients (Kim *et al.*, 2008)

With few exceptions, ginseng appears to be safe if administered within recommended therapeutic doses (WHO, 1999c). *Panax ginseng* reduced the blood concentrations of alcohol and warfarin, and induced mania when used concomitantly with phenelzine, and may increase the efficacy of the influenza vaccination (Hu *et al.*, 2005). While co-administration of ginseng with warfarin does not appear to alter the International Normalized Ratio or platelet aggregation in one clinical trial (Jiang *et al.*, 2005), in another study alterations were observed (Yuan *et al.*, 2004), therefore coadministration of warfaring with ginseng or any herbal medication is not recommended.

4.5.10 *Panax quinquefolius: clinical pharmacology*

Panax quinquefolius L. is the second most important commercial ginseng species and is used somewhat similarly, with the most recent studies showing effi cacy for the prevention of upper respiratory infections, and diabetes, particularly elderly populations.

4.5.11 *Upper respiratory infections*

Three randomized, double-blinded, placebo-controlled clinical trials have assessed the safety and efficacy of a standardized root extract of *P. quinquefolius* containing 80% polysaccharides and 10% protein (Predy *et al.*, 2005). The patients were treated with 400 mg/d of the extract or matching placebo for four months. Ingestion of a polysaccharide-rich extract of the roots of North American ginseng in a moderate dose over four months reduced the mean number of colds per person. The proportion of subjects who experienced two or more colds, the severity of symptoms and the number of days cold symptoms were also reported (Predy *et al.*, 2005).

The other two randomized, double-blind, placebo-controlled clinical trials in investigated the effects of *P. quinquefolius* in institutionalized older adults, average age of 81 and 83 years on acute respiratory illness (ARI) (McElhaney *et al.*, 2004). One eight weeks study, involving 89 volunteers and one 12 weeks study involving 109 subjects, assessed the safety and efficacy of oral administration of 200 mg of *P. quinquefolius* extract twice daily. ARI was defined as two new respiratory symptoms or one with a constitutional symptom. Confirmation of viral ARI was by culture (infl uenza or respiratory syncytial virus (RSV)) or serology for infl uenza. An intent-totreat analysis of pooled data corrected for drug exposure time showed that the incidence of laboratory-confi rmed influenza illness (LCII) was greater in placebo (7 cases/101 subjects) than CVT-E002-treated (1/97) groups (odds ratio (OR) = 7.73, $p = 0.033$). The combined data for LCII and RSV illness were also greater in placebo (9/101) than CVT-E002-treated (1/97) groups (OR = 10.50, $p = 0.009$), for an overall 89% relative risk reduction of ARI in the treatment group. Both studies found that the treatment significantly reduced acute respiratory illnesses associated with infl uenza in older populations with few adverse events (McElhaney *et al.*, 2004).

One review of the randomized controlled trials or controlled clinical trials compared North American (*Panax quinquefolius*) or Asian ginseng (*Panax ginseng*) root extract to placebo or no treatment in healthy adults (Seida *et al.*, 2009). Five trials involving 747 participants were included in the review. Ginseng preparations significantly reduced the total number of common colds by 25% compared to placebo (one trial; 95% CI: 5–45). There was a tendency toward a lower incidence of having at least one common cold or other acute respiratory infection (ARI) in the ginseng group compared to the placebo group (fi ve trials; relative risk: 0.70; 95% CI: 0.48–1.02). Compared to the placebo, ginseng signifi cantly shortened the duration of colds or ARIs by 6.2 days (two trials; 95% CI: 3.4–9.0). The study concluded that *P. quinquefolius* appears to be effective in shortening the duration of colds or ARIs in healthy adults when taken preventatively for durations of 8–16 weeks, but also that more evidence was needed (Seida *et al.*, 2009).

4.5.12 *Diabetes*

Various *P. quinquefolius* extracts, at a dose of 1–3 g have been shown to decrease postprandial glycemia. These data are extensively reviewed and published (WHO, 2009b). In a recent study, the effect of *Panax quinquefolius* saponin (PQS) on blood glucose, blood lipids and insulin sensitivity in patients of coronary heart disease (CHD) with blood glucose abnormality (BGA) was investigated (Zhang *et al.*, 2007). Eighty-four patients with CHD and BGA, as determined by an impaired fasting glucose (IFG), or impaired glucose tolerance (IGT), or type 2 diabetes mellitus (T2DM), were randomly assigned to the PQS group (43 cases) and the control group (41 cases); all were treated with routine Western medicine. The patients in the PQS group were administered PQS orally for four successive weeks in addition to other therapies. Levels of fasting plasma glucose (FPG), fasting insulin (FINS), total cholesterol (TC), triglyceride (TG), high-density lipoprotein cholesterol (HDL-C), low-density lipoprotein cholesterol (LDL-C) were determined both before and after treatment, and insulin sensitive index (ISI) as well as the insulin resistance index and function of beta cells of homostasis model (Homa-IR and Homa-beta) were calculated. FPG decreased in both groups ($p < 0.01$), and the reduction of FPG in the PQS group showed a greater trend (25.80 +/− 12.72) % vs (20.89 +/− 12.17) %, but was not statistically signifi cant. No change in levels of FINS, ISI and Homa-IR was found in either groups ($p > 0.05$). Homa-beta value, which showed insignifi cantly difference before treatment, increased markedly in the PQS group after treatment from 3.48 +/− 0.76 to 4.19 +/− 0.79 ($p < 0.01$), which was higher obviously than the unchanged value of Homa-beta in the control group (3.82 +/− 0.77, $p < 0.05$). There was also a significant decrease of TC and LDL-C levels after treatment in the PQS group ($p < 0.05$), and the TC level in the PQS group (1.17 +/− 0.54) mmol/L was significantly lower than that in the control group [(1.42 +/− 0.49) mmol/L, $p < 0.05$) after treatment.

4.6 Hawthorn

4.6.1 *Introduction*

Hawthorn is the common name of a medicinal plant consisting of the dried whole or cut flower bearing branches of *Crataegus monogyna* Jacq.

(Lindm), *C. laevigata* (Poir.) DC, or related *Crataegus* species of the Rosaceae. Botanically, the genus is complex and members have been classified under different names. *Crataegus laevigata* (Poir.) D.C. has been known synonymously as *Crataegus oxyacantha* L., *C. oxyacantha* L. ssp. *polygala* Lev., *C. oxyacanthoides* Thuill, and *Mespilus oxyacantha* (Gartn.) Crantz; *Crataegus monogyna* Jacq. (Lindm) has the synonyms of: *C. apiifolia* Medik. non Michx., *C. oxyacantha* L. ssp. *monogyna* Lev., *Mespilus elegans* Poir., *M. monogyna* All., and *M. monogyna* Ehrh. *Crataegus* species are thorny shrubs or small trees having bright green, 3–7 lobed leaves and flowers grouped into branchy corymbs having five triangular sepals, five white petals, and an androecium of 15–20 stamens inserted on the receptacle. *Crataegus* species are commonly found in temperate regions, including Asia, Europe and eastern North America and parts of South America (WHO, 2002a; Fong and Bauman, 2002).

4.6.2 Chemistry

Chemically, the major chemical constituents are flavonoids and related proanthocyanidins, with the former being represented by rutin, hyperoside, vitexin, vitexin-2" rhamnoside, acetylvitexin-2" rhamnoside and the latter by the monomeric (−)-epi-catechin and the dimeric procyanidins B-1, -B-2, -B-4, -B-5, -C-1, -D-1, -E and -G. In addition to these phenolic compounds, non-phenolic constituents include the pentacyclic triterpenes ursolic and oleanolic acids, and crataegolic acid. (WHO, 2002a; Fong and Bauman 2002).

4.6.3 Clinical pharmacology

In past years, standardized hydroalcoholic extracts for the treatment of chronic congestive heart failure stage II, as defined by the New York Heart Association have been investigated, and detailed reviews of the outcomes of these clinical trials are published (Fong and Bauman 2002; Pilter *et al.*, 2009; WHO, 2002a; UNESCO, 2007). While previous studies reported positive assessments for the use of Hawthorn extracts for the management of cardiovascular disease (Pilter *et al.*, 2009), more recent studies have reported negative results (Zick *et al.*, 2009; Holubarsch *et al.*, 2009).

4.6.4 *Chronic heart failure*

Hydroalcoholic extracts of hawthorn extract are advocated as an oral treatment for chronic heart failure, and the German Commission E has approved the use of extracts of hawthorn leaf with flower in patients suffering from heart failure graded stage II according to the New York Heart Association (Pilter *et al.*, 2008). The most recent Cochrane assessment of hawthorn reviewed 14 randomized, double-blind, and placebo controlled trials that used hawthorn leaf and flower extract monopreparations (Pilter *et al.*, 2008). Fourteen trials met all inclusion criteria and were included in the review. In most of the clinical trials, hawthorn was used as an adjunct therapy to conventional treatment. Ten trials including 855 patients with chronic heart failure (New York Heart Association classes I to III) provided data for the meta-analysis. Overall for the outcomes of increased workload, treatment with hawthorn extract was more benefi cial than placebo (WMD (Watt) 5.35, 95% CI 0.71 to 10.00, $p < 0.02$, $n = 380$), also exercise tolerance also significantly increased after treatment with hawthorn extract (WMD (Watt x min) 122.76, 95% CI 32.74 to 212.78, $n = 98$). In addition, the pressure-heart rate product, an index of cardiac oxygen consumption, showed a beneficial decrease after hawthorn treatment (WMD (mmHg/min) -19.22, 95% CI -30.46 to -7.98, $n = 264$). Symptoms such as shortness of breath and fatigue were significantly improved with hawthorn treatment as compared with placebo (WMD -5.47, 95% CI -8.68 to -2.26, $n = 239$). No data on relevant mortality and morbidity such as cardiac events wwwere reported, apart from one trial, which reported deaths (three in active, one in control) without providing further details. Reported adverse events were infrequent, mild, and transient; they includ]ed nausea, dizziness, and cardiac and gastrointestinal complaints. These results suggest that there is a signifi cant benefi t in from hawthorn extract as an adjunctive treatment for chronic heart failure (Pilter *et al.*, 2008).

However, more recently, a randomized, double-blind, placebo-controlled trial involving 120 ambulatory patients aged ≥ 18 years with

New York Heart Association (NYHA) class II-III chronic heart failure assessed the effects of hawthorn therapy as adjunct to conventional treatment (Zick *et al.*, 2009). All patients received conventional medical therapy, as tolerated, and were randomized to either hawthorn 450 mg twice daily or placebo for six months (Zick *et al.*, 2009). The primary outcome was change in six mins walking distance (exercise tolerance) at six months. Secondary outcomes included quality of life (QOL) measures, peak oxygen consumption, and anaerobic threshold during maximal treadmill exercise testing, NYHA classification, left ventricular ejection fraction (LVEF), neurohormones, and measures of oxidative stress and infl ammation. The results of the study showed were no signifi cant differences between the hawthorn or placebo groups in the change in six mins walk distance ($p = 0.61$), or on measures of QOL, functional capacity, neurohormones, oxidative stress, or infl ammation after six months of therapy. There were significantly more adverse events reported in the hawthorn group ($p = 0.02$), although most were non-cardiac. This study concluded that adjunct therapy with a hawthorn extract provides no symptomatic or functional benefit when given with standard medical therapy to patients with heart failure.

In a second study published in 2009 (SPICE study), data on the efficacy and safety of hawthorn extracts as an add-on treatment for congestive heart failure, in a large morbidity/mortality trial was investigated in a large clinical study (Holubarsch *et al.*, 2008). The *Crataegus* extract WS 1442 was used in this randomized, double-blind, placebo-controlled multicenter study, involving 2681 adults (WS 1442: 1338; placebo: 1343) with NYHA class II or III CHF and reduced left ventricular ejection fraction (LVEF $\geq$ 35%) were included and received 900 mg/day WS 1442 or placebo for 24 months. Primary endpoint was time until first cardiac event. The results showed that the average time to first cardiac event was 620 days for WS 1442 and 606 days for placebo (event rates: 27.9% and 28.9%, hazard ratio (HR): 0.95, 95% CI [0.82;1.10]; $p = 0.476$). The trend for cardiac mortality reduction with WS 1442 (9.7% at month 24; HR: 0.89 [0.73;1.09]) was not statistically signifi cant ($p = 0.269$). In the subgroup with LVEF $\geq$ 25%, WS 1442 reduced sudden cardiac death by 39.7% (HR 0.59 [0.37;0.94] at month 24; $p = 0.025$). Adverse events were comparable in both groups.

Thus this study concluded that treatment with WS 1442 had no signifi cant effect on the primary endpoint (time until fi rst cardiac event). WS 1442 was safe to use in patients receiving optimal medication for heart failure. However, the data also suggested that WS 1442 may reduce the incidence of sudden cardiac death, in patients with less compromised left ventricular function and thus this is worthy of further investigation (Holubarsch *et al.*, 2008).

4.7 Huperzia

4.7.1 *Introduction*

Chinese club moss is the whole plant of *Huperzia serrata* (Thunb. ex Murray) Trev. [syn. *Lycopodium serratum* Thunb. ex Murray) of the family Huperziaceae. The whole plant body is used in traditional Chinese medicine as *"Qian Ceng Ta"* for over 1000 years in China for the treatment of a number of ailments, including contusions, strains, swellings, schizophrenia, rheumatism, blood circulation, colds, and myasthenia gravis (College, 1985; Ma, 1997). The significance of this medicinal plant was not apparent globally until the discovery of huperzine A, one of its chemical constituents, as a potential therapeutic agent in the management of Alzheimer's disease (Liu *et al.*, 1986a; 1986b).

For the purpose of the present discussion on *"Botanical Supplements for Aging"*, we have strived to concentrate on herbal materials that have been subjected to clinical evaluation, rather than one of its chemical constituents as in the case of *Huperzia serrata*, for which the compound huperzine A was the subject of clinical studies. However, given the fact that Alzheimer's disease affects so many elderly people and the fact that in addition to the use of huperzine in clinical therapy, there is available in China, a commercial product containing extracts of *Huperzia serrata*, rich in huperzine, in the form of a tablet (*"Shuangyiping"*) as a drug for symptomatic treatment of AD in China (Tang, 1996). Further, powdered *Huperzia serrata*, in tablet or capsule forms, are also marketed in the USA as a dietary supplement for the same purpose. Hence, *Huperzia serrata* is included in this chapter, with discussions on the biological/clinical aspects being devoted to the active compound, huperzine A.

Huperzia serrata, like other members of the Huperzia, is a terrestrial and erect plant, with gemmae present, and fertile leaves being normally the same size as sterile leaves and sporophytes reaching a height of 5–15 cm. Members of the genus Huperzia are widely distributed in tropical, subtropical, and temperate zones in China. Although H. serrata is the only relatively common Huperziaceae species distributed in China, it is not abundantly found and grows very slowly, requiring 15–20 years of growth from spore germination to maturity in very specialized habitats. Because of the high demand for huperzine A and the marketing of H. serrata extracts as a drug as well as a dietary supplement, wild populations of H. serrata and related species may soon be decimated (Ma and Gang, 2004; Ma *et al.*, 2006).

4.7.2 *Chemistry*

Chemically, the biologically active huperzine A was the first of more than 50 lycopodium alkaloids isolated from *H. serrata* at a concentration of *ca.* 0.007% (Liu *et al.*, 1986a). Subsequently, huperzines B, -C, -D, -E, -F, -G, -H, -I, -J, -K, -L, -M,-N, -O, -P, -Q, -R,-S, -T, -U, -V, and -W, and some 30 other lycopodium alkaloids of a variety of structural complexity have been reported from this plant (Ma *et al.*, 2007).

4.7.3 *Clinical pharmacology*

The clinical pharmacology will focus on huperzine A, as it is the active constituent of Huperzia, and there are no randomized controlled clinical studies for the plant extract. Hyperzine A has been used in the management of the symptoms of Alzheimer disease (AD) (Desilets *et al.*, 2009; Little *et al.*, 2008, Li *et al.*, 2008; Ma *et al.*, 2006; 2007; Tang *et al.*, 1996). One of the pathways by which AD induces symptoms is via the degeneration of acetylcholine-containing neurons in the basal forebrain. Thus, cholinesterase inhibitors that block the degradation of acetylcholine may increase the efficacy of the cholinergic neurons, thereby reducing the symptoms of AD (Desilets *et al.*, 2009; Little *et al.*, 2008).

4.7.4 *Alzheimer disease*

Huperzine A is a linearly competitive, reversible inhibitor of acetyl cholinesterase that has both central and peripheral activity with the ability to protect cells against hydrogen peroxide, beta-amyloid protein (or peptide), glutamate, ischemia and staurosporine-induced cytotoxicity and apoptosis (Li *et al.*, 2008; Little *et al.*, 2008). One meta-analysis has reviewed randomized controlled clinical trials (RCTs), to assess the safety and effi cacy of huperzine A for the treatment of patients with AD (Li *et al.*, 2008). Six clinical trials involving 454 patients met the inclusion criteria, however, the methodological quality of most included trials was low. Huperzine A had beneficial effects on the improvement of general cognitive function measured by MMSE (WMD 2.81; 95% CI, $p < 0.00001$) and ADAS-Cog at six weeks (WMD 1.91; 95% CI) and at 12 weeks (WMD 2.51; 95% CI), global clinical assessment measured by CDR (WMD −0.80; 95% CI) and CIBIC-plus (OR 4.32, 95% CI), behavioral disturbance measured by ADAS-non-Cog at six weeks (WMD −1.33, 95% CI) and at 12 weeks (WMD −1.52, 95% CI), and functional performance measured by ADL (WMD = −7.17; 95% CI; $p < 0.00001$), as compared with placebo. However, huperzine A was not superior to placebo in the improvement of general cognitive function measured by Hasegawa Dementia Scale (HDS) (WMD: 2.78; 95% CI, $p = 0.06$) and specific cognitive function measured by Weshler Memory Scale (WMS) (WMD = 6.64; 95% CI; $p = 0.19$). There were no significant differences in adverse events between huperzine A and placebo. This meta-analysis concludes that huperzine A seems to have some beneficial effects on the improvement of general cognitive function, global clinical status, behavioral disturbance and functional performance, with no obvious serious adverse events for patients with AD. However, poor study quality makes recommendations diffi cult, and larger, more rigorous randomized, multi-center, trials for huperzine A for AD are needed (Li *et al.*, 2008).

4.8 Pygeum

4.8.1 *Introduction*

Pygeum, or African prune, is an herbal product consisting of the dried bark of the trunk of *Prunus africana* (Hook. f.) Kalkman (Rosaceae) (WHO, 2002b).

Products containing Pygeum are used for the treatment of benign prostatic hyperplasia (BPH) (WHO, 2002b). The plant is an evergreen tree, usually 10–25m high, with straight, cylindrical trunk and dense, rounded crown. Leaves alternate, 8–12cm long, long-stalked, simple, elliptic, bluntly pointed at apex, with shallow crenate margins; leathery, deep green and glossy, with midrib sharply impressed or channeled on upper surface and strongly prominent on underside; smell of almonds when bruised. The dried trunk bark is red to blackish-brown, deeply square-fissured or corrugated (Bruneton, 1995; Beentje, 1994; Van Breitenbach, 1974). It is found in mountain forests of equatorial Africa, including Angola, Cameroon, Ethiopia, Ghana, Kenya, Madagascar, Malawi, Mozambique, Republic of Congo, South Africa, Uganda, United Republic of Tanzania, Zambia and Zimbabwe (Bombardelli and Morazzoni, 1997; Beentje, 1994, Van Breitenbach 1974).

4.8.2 Chemistry

Chemically, the purported active constituents include docosanol (0.6%) and b-sitosterol (15.7%). Other major constituents include alkanols (tetracosanol [0.5%] and trans-ferulic acid esters of docosanol and tetracosanol), fatty acids (62.3%, comprising myristic, palmitic, linoleic, oleic, stearic, arachidic, behenic and lignoceric acids); sterols (sitosterone [2.0%] and daucosterol) and triterpenes (ursolic acid [2.9%], friedelin [1.4%], 2-a-hydroxyursolic acid [0.5%], epimaslinic acid [0.8%] and maslinic acid) (Bombardelli and Morazzoni, 1997; Martinelli, 1986; Pierini et al., 1982; Uberti E et al., 1990; Catalano et al., 1984; Longo and Tira, 1981; 1983; Nieri E et al., 1996).

4.8.3 Clinical pharmacology

Benign Prostatic Hyperplasia

Pygeum africanum, is one of the several phytotherapeutic agents available for the treatment of Benign Prostatic Hyperplasia (BPH) (Edgar et al., 2007; Wilt et al., 2002; WHO, 2002b). A systematic review of the clinical trials assessed if the evidence for extracts of Pygeum africanum supporting its use in the treatment of BPH are as effective as standard pharmacologic BPH treatments and have fewer adverse events as compared with standard

BPH drugs. The main outcome measure for comparing the effectiveness of *Pygeum africanum* with placebo and standard BPH medications was the change in urologic symptoms scale scores. Secondary outcomes included change in urologic symptoms including nocturia and urodynamic measures (peak and mean urine flow, prostate size). The main outcome measure for adverse effects was the number of men reporting adverse effects. A total of 18 randomized controlled trials involving 1562 men met inclusion criteria and were analyzed (Wilt *et al.*, 2002). Only one of the studies reported a method of treatment allocation concealment, though 17 were double-blinded. There were no studies comparing *Pygeum africanum* to standard pharmacologic interventions such as alpha-adrenergic blockers or 5-alpha reductase inhibitors. The mean study duration was 64 days (range, 30–122 days). Compared to men receiving placebo, *Pygeum africanum* provided a moderately large improvement in the combined outcome of urologic symptoms and flow measures as assessed by an effect size defined by the difference of the mean change for each outcome divided by the pooled standard deviation for each outcome (−0.8 SD [95% confidence interval (CI), −1.4, −0.3 (n = 6 studies)]). Men using *Pygeum africanum* were more than twice as likely to report an improvement in overall symptoms (RR = 2.1, 95% CI = 1.4, 3.1). Nocturia was reduced by 19%, residual urine volume by 24% and peak urine flow was increased by 23%. Adverse effects due to *P. africanum* were mild and comparable to placebo. The overall dropout rate was 12% and was similar between *Pygeum africanum* (13%), placebo (11%) and other controls (8%). The review concluded that a standardized preparation of *Pygeum africanum* may be a useful treatment option for men with lower urinary symptoms consistent with benign prostatic hyperplasia. However, the reviewed studies were small in size, were of short duration, used varied doses and preparations and rarely reported outcomes using standardized validated measures of effi cacy (Wilt *et al.*, 2002).

4.9 Saw Palmetto

4.9.1 *Introduction*

Saw Palmetto is the common name of a botanical reputed to have beneficial effects for alleviating benign prostatic hyperplasia in men. It consist of the dried ripe fruits of *Serenoa repens* (Bartr.) Small. (Aracaceae) (Blumenthal *et al.*, 1998; USP, 1999; WHO, 2002c). The plant is a low scrubby palm growing in sandy soil, with characteristic creeping rhizome, one end of which rises a short distance above ground, surrounded by a dense crown of leaves with saw-like margins. The petioles are slender and spinose on edges; the blade fan-shaped, with palmate divisions that are slightly cleft at the summit; the inflorescence is densely tomentose and shorter than the leaves; and the fruit is a single seeded drupe (Gathercoal and Wirth, 1936), which is superior, ellipsoidal, ovoid or somewhat globular, 1.5–3.0 cm long, 1.0– 1.5 cm in diameter; dark brown to black with a smooth, dull surface, somewhat oily, with a few large, angular depressions and ridges. This plant is indigenous to the South-East of the United States of America, from South Carolina to Florida (Gathercoal and Wirth, 1936).

4.9.2 Chemistry

Chemically, the major constituents are free fatty acids and their corresponding ethyl esters; sterols and lipids. The primary fatty acid constituents include oleic, lauric, myristic, palmitic, linoleic, caphoic, caprylic, capric, palmitoleic, stearic and linolenic acids (Farnsworth, 2009; De Swaef and Vlietinck, 1996; Wajda-Dubois, 1996). The major sterols include ß- sitosterol, stigmasterol and daucosterol (Hänsel R *et al.*, 1964). The lipids consist of triglycerides of fatty acids.

4.9.3 *Clinical pharmacology*

Benign Prostatic Hyperplasia

Extracts of saw palmetto are used for the management of the symptoms of benign prostatic hyperplasia (BPH), a non-malignant enlargement of the prostate, causing obstructive and irritative lower urinary tract symptoms (LUTS) (Tacklind *et al.*, 2009; WHO, 2002c). A recent systematic review assessed the effi cacy of *Serenoa repens* in the treatment of LUTS consistent with BPH (Tacklind *et al.*, 2009). The main outcome measured for comparing the effectiveness of *Serenoa repens* with placebo or other interventions was the change in urologic symptom-scale scores.

Secondary outcomes included changes in nocturia and urodynamic measures. The main outcome measure for side effects or adverse events was the number of men reporting side effects. Nine new trials involving 2053 men (a 64.8% increase), for the main comparison — *Serenoa repens* versus placebo — three trials were included with 419 subjects and three endpoints (IPSS, peak urine flow, prostate size). Overall, 5222 subjects from 30 randomized trials lasting from four to 60 weeks were assessed. Twenty-six trials were double-blinded and treatment allocation concealment was adequate in eighteen studies. *Serenoa repens* was not superior to placebo in improving IPSS urinary symptom scores, (WMD (weighted mean difference) -0.77 points, 95% CI -2.88 to 1.34, $p > 0.05$; two trials), finasteride (MD (mean difference) 0.40 points, 95% CI -0.57 to 1.37, $p > 0.05$; one trial), or tamsulosin (WMD -0.52 points, 95% CI -1.91 to 0.88, $p > 0.05$; two trials). For nocturia, *Serenoa repens* was significantly better than placebo (WMD -0.78 nocturnal visits, 95% CI -1.34 to -0.22, $p < 0.05$; nine trials), but with the caveat of significant heterogeneity ($I(2) = 66\%$). A sensitivity analysis, utilizing higher quality, larger trials (≥ 40 subjects), demonstrated no signifi cant difference (WMD -0.31 nocturnal visits, 95% CI -0.70 to 0.08, $p > 0.05$; fi ve trials) ($I(2) = 11\%$). *Serenoa repens* was not superior to finasteride (MD -0.05 nocturnal visits, 95% CI -0.49 to 0.39, $p > 0.05$; one trial), or to tamsulosin (% improvement) (RR) (risk ratio) 0.91, 95% CI 0.66 to 1.27, $p > 0.05$; one trial). Comparing peak urine fl ow, *Serenoa repens* was not superior to placebo at trial endpoint (WMD 1.02 ml/s, 95% CI -0.14 to 2.19, $p > 0.05$; ten trials), or by comparing mean change (WMD 0.31 ml/s, 95% CI -0.56 to 1.17, $p > 0.05$; two trials). Comparing prostate size at endpoint, there was no signifi cant difference between *Serenoa repens* and placebo (MD -1.05 cc, 95% CI -8.84 to 6.75, $p > 0.05$; two trials), or by comparing mean change (MD -1.22 cc, 95% CI -3.91 to 1.47, $p > 0.05$; one trial). The review concluded that based on the current evidence, saw palmetto is not more effective than placebo for the management of LUTS associated with BPH (Tacklind *et al.*, 2009).

Adverse events associated with the use of *S. repens* are mild and similar to those with placebo (Agbabiaka *et al.*, 2009). The most frequently reported adverse events are abdominal pain, diarrhoea, nausea, fatigue, headache, decreased libido and rhinitis. More serious adverse events such as death and cerebral hemorrhage are reported in isolated case reports and data from spontaneous reporting schemes, but causality is questionable. No drug interactions were reported.

4.10 Conclusions

Demographic indicators suggest that expanding aging populations with continuing need for medical services will continue to increase in all countries. As such, it is reasonable to predict that specific interest in and use of CAM modalities, including botanicals, will expand as well. The list of botanicals with potential benefit for aging populations is increasing, however, rigorous clinical trials assessing quality, safety and effi cacy are still urgently needed. In addition, drug interaction studies will also play an important role in addressing the needs of the elderly. Since this population has the highest rate of chronic disease and prescription drug use, the potential impact of botanical-drug interactions is a signifi cant question that still has not been adequately addressed.

References

Agbabiaka, T.B., Pittle, M.H., Wider, B. and Ernst, E. (2009) *Serenoa repens* (saw palmetto): A systematic review of adverse events. *Drug Saf.* **32**, 637–647.

Anon. (2000) *Database on Medicinal Plants used in Ayurveda.* New Delhi, Central Council for Research in Ayurveda and Siddha, Department of ISM and H, Ministry of Health and Family Welfare, Government of India.

Assinewe, V.A., Baum, B.R., Gagnon, D. and Arnason, J.T. (2003) Phytochemistry of wild populatrions of *Panax quinquefolius* L. (North American ginseng). *J. Agr. Food Chem.* **57**, 4549–4553.

Astin, J.A., Pelletier, K.R., Marie, A. and Haskell, W.L. (2000) Complementary and alternative medicine use among elderly persons: One-year analysis of a Blue Shield Medicare supplement. *J. Gerontol. A. Biol. Sci. Med. Sci.* **55**, M4–M9.

Awang, D.V.C. (2000) The neglected ginsenosides of North American ginseng (*Panax quinquefolius* L.). *J. Herbs. Spices. Med. Plants* **7**, 103–109. Awang, D. (2003) What in the name of Panax are those other "Ginsengs"? *HerbalGram* **57**, 35–40.

Ayurvedic Pharmacopoeia of India, Part I, Vol. IV. Ministry of Health and Family Welfare, New Delhi, Department of Indian System of Medicine and Homeopathy. (1999). Barnes, P.M. and Bloom, B. (2008) Complementary and alternative medicine use Among adults and children in the United States, 2007. *Nat. Health Stat. Reports* **12**, 1–24.

Barnes, P.M., Powell-Griner, E. and McFann, K. (2004) Complementary and alternative medicine use among adults: United States, 2002. Advance data from the Vital and Health Statistics; No. 343. Hyattsville, MD: National Center for Health Statistics.

Beentje, H. (1994) *Kenyan Trees, Shrubs and Lianas.* Nairobi, National Museums of Kenya. Birks, J. and Grimley, E.J. (2009) *Ginkgo biloba* for cognitive impairment and dementia. *Cochrane Database Syst Rev.* (1): CD003120. Blumenthal, M., Busse, W.R., Goldberg, A. *et al.,* (eds.) (1998) *The Complete German Commission E Monographs.* American Botanical Council, Austin, TX.

Bombardelli, E. and Morazzoni, P. (1997) *Prunus africana* (Hook. f) Kalkm. *Fitoterapia.* **68**, 205–218.

Brownie, S. (2006) Why are elderly individuals at risk of nutritional defi ciency? *Int. J. Nurs. Pract.* **12**, 110–118.

Bruneton, J. (1995) *Pharmacognosy, Phytochemistry, Medicinal Plants.* Paris, Lavoisier.

Catalano, S., *et al.* (1984) New constituents of *Prunus africana* bark extract. *J. Nat. Prod.* **47**, 910.

Cui, J.F. (1995) Identification and quantification of ginsenosides in various commercial ginseng preparations. *Eur. J. Pharm. Sci.* **3**, 77–85.

College, J.N.M. (1985) *The Dictionary of Traditional Chinese Medicine.* Shanghai Sci-Tech Press, Shanghai.

DeFeudis, F.V. (1991) *Ginkgo Biloba Extract (EGb 761): Pharmacological Activities and Clinical Applications.* Editions, Elsevier, Paris. Scientifi ques.

DeKosky, S.T., Williamson, J.D., Fitzpatrick, A.L., Kronmal, R.A., Ives, D.G., Saxton, J.A., Lopez, O.L., Burke, G., Carlson, M.C., Fried, L.P., Kuller, L.H., Robbins, J.A., Tracy, R.P., Woolard, N.F., Dunn, L., Snitz, B.E., Nahin, R.L., Furberg, C.D and Ginkgo Evaluation of Memory (GEM) Study Investigators. (2008) *Ginkgo biloba* for prevention of dementia: A randomized controlled trial. *J. Am. Med. Assoc.* **300**, 2253–2262.

Desilets, A.R., Gickas, J.J. and Dunican, K.C. (2009) Role of huperzine A in the treatment of Alzheimer's disease. *Ann Pharmacother.* **43**, 514–518.

De Swaef, S.I. and Vlietinck, A.J. (1996) Simultaneous quantitation of lauric acid and ethyl laureate in *Sabal serrulata* by capillary gas chromatography and derivatisation with trimethylsulphonium hydroxide. *J. Chromatogr.* **719**, 479–482.

Edgar, A.D., Levin, R., Constantinou, C.E. and Denis, L. (2007) A critical review of the pharmacology of the plant extract of *Pygeum africanum* in the treatment of LUTS. *Neurourol Urodyn.* **26**, 458–463.

Ernst, E. (2008) Frankincense: A systematic review. *Brit. Med. J.* **337**, 2813.

Girgune, J.B. and Garg, B.D. (1979) Chemical investigation of the essential oil from *Boswellia serrata* Roxb. *J. Sci. Res.* **1**, 119–122.

Farnsworth, N.R. (ed.) (2009) *NAPRALERT Database.* http://www.napralert.org/. University of Illinois at Chicago, Chicago, Chicago, IL.

Fong, H.H.S. and Bauman, J.L. (2002) Hawthorn. *J. Card. Nurs.* **16**(4), 1–8.

Gathercoal, E.N. and Wirth, E.H. (1936) *Pharmacognosy.* Lea & Febiger, Philadelphia.

Gupta, I., *et al.* (1998) Effects of *Boswellia serrata* gum resin in patients with bronchial asthma: Results of a double-blind, placebo-controlled, 6-week clinical study. *Eur. J. Med. Res* **3**, 511–514.

Gupta, I., *et al.* (1997) Effects of *Boswellia serrata* gum resin in patients with ulcerative colitis. *Eur. J. Med. Res.* **21**, 37–43. Gupta, I., *et al.*, (2001) Effects of gum resin of *Boswellia serrata* in patients with chronic colitis. *Planta Medica.* **67**, 391–395.

Hänsel, R., *et al.* (1964) Eine Dünnschichtchromatographische Untersuchung der Sabalfrüchte. *Planta Med.* **12**, 136–139.

Hänsel, R. *et al.* (eds.) (1994) *Hagers Handbuch der Pharmazeutischen Praxis*, Vol. 6, 5th edn. Springer-Verlag Berlin.

Heo, J.H., Lee, S.T., Chu, K., Oh, M.J., Park, H.J., Shim, J.Y. and Kim, M. (2008) An open-label trial of Korean red ginseng as an adjuvant treatment for cognitive impairment in patients with Alzheimer's disease. *Eur. J. Neurol.* **15**, 865–868.

HKCMMS (2009) *Hong Kong Chinese Materia Medica Standards*, Vol. 3. Dept of Health, Hong Kong Special Administrative Region, The People's Republic of China.

Holubarsch, C.J., Colucci, W.S., Meinertz, T., Gaus, W. and Tendera, M. (2008) The efficacy and safety of *Crataegus* extract WS 1442 in patients with heart failure: The SPICE trial. *Eur. J. Heart Fail.* **10**, 1255–1263.

Hu, S.Y. (1976) The genus *Panax* (ginseng) in Chinese medicine. *Econ. Bot.* **30**, 11–28.

Huh, H. and Staba, E.J. (1992) The botany and chemistry of *Ginkgo biloba* L. *J. Herbs Spices Med. Plants.* **1**, 91–124.

Humpel, N. and Jones, S.C. (2006) Gaining insight into the what, why, and where of complementary and alternative medicine use by cancer patients and survivors. *Eur. J. Cancer Care.* **15**, 362–368.

Jang, D.J., Lee, M.S., Shin, B.C., Lee, Y.C. and Ernst, E. (2008) Red ginseng for treating erectile dysfunction: A systematic review. *Br. J. Clin. Pharmacol.* **66**, 444–450.

Kapoor, VK, Dureja J, and Chadha R. (2009) Herbals in the control of ageing. *Drug Discov. Today* **14**(19–20), 992–998.

Kapoor, L.D. *(1990) Handbook of Ayurvedic Medicinal Plants.* CRC Press, Boca Raton.

Kasper, S, and Schubert, H. (2009) [*Ginkgo biloba* extract EGb 761 in the treatment of dementia: evidence of efficacy and tolerability][Article in German]. *Fortschr Neurol Psychiatr* **77**, 494–506.

Keys, J.D. (1976) *Chinese Herbs, their Botany, Chemistry and Pharmacodynamics.* CE Tuttle, Rutland,VT.

Kimmatkar, N. (2003) Efficacy and tolerability of *Boswellia serrata* extract in treatment of osteoarthritis of knee — a randomized double blind placebo controlled trial. *Phytomedicine* **10**, 3–7.

Kim, T.H., Jeon, S.H., Hahn, E.J., Paek, K.Y., Park, J.K., Youn, N.Y. and Lee, H.L. (2009) Effects of tissue-cultured mountain ginseng (*Panax ginseng* CA Meyer) extract on male patients with erectile dysfunction. *Asian J. Androl.* **11**, 356–361.

Lee, S.T., Chu, K., Sim, J.Y., Heo, J.H. and Kim, M. (2008) *Panax ginseng* enhances cognitive performance in Alzheimer disease. *Alzheimer Dis. Assoc. Disord.* **22**, 222–226.

Linde, K., Barrett, B., Wölkart, K., Bauer, R. and Melchart, D. (2006) *Echinacea* for preventing and treating the common cold. *Cochrane Database Syst. Rev.* (1): CD000530.

List, P.H., Horhamme, L. (eds.) (1975) *Hagers Handbuch der Pharmazeutischen Praxis*, 4th ed., Springer Verlag Berlin.

Li, J., Wu, H.M., Zhou, R.L., Liu, G.J. and Dong, B.R. (2008) Huperzine A for Alzheimer's disease. *Cochrane Database Syst Rev.* (2): CD005592.

Little, J.T., Walsh, S. and Aisen, P.S. (2008) An update on huperzine A as a treatment for Alzheimer's disease. *Expert Opin. Investig. Drugs* **17**, 209–215.

Liu, J.S., Yu, C.M., Zhou, Y.Z., Han, Y.Y., Wu, F.W., Qi, B.F. and Zhu, Y.L. (1986a). Study on the chemistry of huperzine-A and huperzine-B. *Acta Chim. Sinica.* **44**, 1035–1040.

Liu, J.S., Zhu, Y.L., Yu, C.M., Zhou, Y.Z., Han, Y.Y., Wu, F.W. and Qi, B.F. (1986b). The structures of huperzine A and B, two new alkaloids exhibiting marked anticholinesterase activity. *Can. J. Chem.* **64**, 837–839.

Longo, R. and Tira, S. (1981) Constituents of *Pygeum africanum* bark. *Planta Med.* **42**, 195–203.

Longo, R. and Tira, S. (1983) Steroidal and other components of *Pygeum africanum* bark. *Il Farmaco.* **38**, 287–292.

Ma, X.Q. (1997) Chemical Studies on Natural Resources of *Huperzia* and Its Related Genera in China. *Chinese Acad. Sci. [D]*, Shanghai.

Ma, X. and Gang, D.R. (2004) The *Lycopodium* alkaloids. *Nat. Prod. Rept* **21**, 752–772.

Ma, X., Tan, C., Zhu, D. and Gang, D.R. (2006) A survey of potential huperzine A natural resources in China: The Huperziaceae. *J. Ethnopharmacol.* **104**, 54–67.

Ma, X., Tan, C., Zhu, D., Gang, D.R. and Xiao, P. (2007) Huperzine A from *Huperzia* species — an ethnopharmacolgical review. *J. Ethnopharmacol.* **113**, 15–34.

Mahady, G.B., Fong, H.H.S. and Farnsworth, N.R. (2001a) *Botanical Dietary Supplements: Quality, Safety and Efficacy.* Swets & Zeitlinger Publishers, Lisse, The Netherlands.

Mahady, G.B., Qato, D.M., Gyllenhaal, C.G., Chadwick, L. and Fong, H.H.S. (2001b) *Echinacea*: Recommendations for its use in prophylaxis and treatment of respiratory tract infections. *Nutr. Clin. Care.* **4**(4), 199–208.

Mahady, G.B. (2007) Medicinal plants for the prevention and treatment of coronary heart disease. In: *Encyclopedia* of Life Support Systems (EOLSS) *Ethnopharmacology* (eds.) Elizabethsky, E. and Etikin, N., UNESCO Publishing-Eolss Publishers, Oxford, UK.

McElhaney, J.E., Gravenstein, S., Cole S.K., Davidson, E., O'neill, D., Petitjean, S., Rumble, B. and Shan, J.J. (2004). A placebo-controlled trial of a proprietary extract of North American ginseng (CVT-E002) to prevent acute respiratory illness in institutionalized older adults. *J. Am. Geriatr. Soc.* **52**(1), 13–19.

Martinelli, E.M., Seraglia, R. and Pifferi, G. (1986) Characterization of *Pygeum africanum* bark extracts by HRGC with computer assistance. *J. High Res. Chromatogr. Commun.* **9**, 106–110.

Nadkarni, K.M. (1954) *Indian Material Medica.* Popular Prakashan Bombay.

National Center for Health Statistics, Centers for Disease Control and Prevention. (2008) http://www.cdc.gov/nchs/pressroom/97facts/disable.htm. Accessed July 22, 2008.

Nieri, E. *et al.* (1996) New lignans from *Prunus africanum* Hook. *Rivista Ital. Eppos.* **7** 27–31.

Oshima, Y., Sato, K. and Hikino, H. (1987) Isolation and hypoglycemic activity of quinque-folans A, B, and C, glycans of *Panax quinquefolium* roots. *J. Nat. Prod.* **50**, 188–190.

Pharmacopoeia Commission. (1992) *Pharmacopoeia of the People's Republic of China* (English ed.) Science and Technology Press. Guangzhou, Guangdong.

Pierini, N. *et al.* (1982) Identification and determination of N-docosanol in the bark extract of *Pygeum africanum* and in patent medicines containing it. *Boll. Chim. Farm.* **121**, 27–34.

Pittler, M.H, and Ernst E. (2008) Hawthorn extract for treating chronic heart failure. *Cochrane Database Syst. Rev.* **23**(1): CD005312.

Predy, G.N., Goel, V., Lovlin, R., Donner, A., Stitt, L. and Basu, T.K. (2005) Efficacy of an extract of North American ginseng containing poly-furanosyl-pyranosyl-saccharides for preventing upper respiratory tract infections: a randomized controlled trial. *Can. Med.Assoc. J.* **173**, 1043–1048.

Sabbagh, M.N. (2009) Drug development for Alzheimer's disease: Where are we now and where are we headed? *Am. J. Geriatr. Pharmacother.* **7**, 167–185.

Sander, O. Herborn, G. and Rau, R. (1998) Is H15 (resin extract of *Boswellia serrata*, "incense") a useful supplement to establish drug therapy of chronic polyarthritis? Results of a double-blind pilot study. *Zeitschrift fur Rheumatologie.* **57**, 11–16.

Sebastian, R.S., Cleveland, L.E., Goldman, J.D. and Moshfegh, A.J. (2007) Older adults who use vitamin/mineral supplements differ from nonusers in nutrient intake adequacy and dietary attitudes. *J. Am. Diet. Assoc.* **107**, 1322–1332.

Seida, J.K., Durec, T. and Kuhle, S. (2009) North American (*Panax quinquefolius*) and Asian Ginseng (*Panax ginseng*) preparations for prevention of the common cold in healthy adults: A systematic review. *Evid Based Complement Alternat Med.* doi: 10.1093/ecam/ne p. 068.

Shah, S.A., Sander, S., White, C.M., Rinaldi, M. and Coleman, C.I. (2007) Evaluation of *echinacea* for the prevention and treatment of the common cold: A meta-analysis. *Lancet Infect. Dis.* **7**, 473–480.

Shibata, S., Tanaka, O., Shoji, J. and Saito, H. (1985) Chemistry and pharmacology of panax. In: *Economic and Medicinal Plants Research*, Vol. 1. (eds.) Wagner, H. and Farnsworth, N.R. Academic Press, London pp. 217–284.

Singh, G.B., Bani, S. and Singh, S. (1996) Toxicity and safety evaluation of *Boswellic* acids. *Phytomedicine* **3**, 87–90.

Sprecher, E. (1987) Ginseng — Miracle drug or phytopharmacon? *Deutsche Apotheker Zeitung.* **9**, 52–61.

Sticher, O. (1994) Biochemical, pharmaceutical and medical perspectives of *Ginkgo* preparations. In: *New Drug Development from Herbal Medicines in Neuropsychopharmacology.* Symposium of the XIXth CINP Congress, Washington, DC, June 27–July 1, 1994.

Sticher, O. (1993) Quality of *Ginkgo* preparations. *Planta Med.* **59**, 2–11.

Tacklind J., MacDonald R., Rutks I. and Wilt T.J. (2009) *Serenoa repens* for benign prostatic hyperplasia. *Cochrane Database Syst Rev.* (2):CD001423.

Tang, X.C. (1996) Huperzine A shuangyiping: A promising drug for Alzheimer's disease. *Zhongguo Yao Li Xue Bao.* **17**, 481–484.

Tyler, V.E., Brady, L.R. and Robbers, J.E. (1981) *Pharmacognosy.* Lea and Febiger, Philadelphia.

Uberti, E., *et al.*, (1990) HPLC analysis of N-docosyl ferulate in *Pygeum africanum* extracts and pharmaceutical formulations. *Fitoterapia.* **61**, 342–347.

U.S. Department of Health and Human Services (2000) Washington, DC: USDHHS Healthy People 2010.

United States Pharmacopoeia Countries (1999) *The United States Pharmacopoeia 24: National Formulary 19.* Pharmacopoeial Convention. Rockville, MD, United States.

Van Breitenbach, F. (1974) *Southern Cape Forests and Trees.* Government Printers for the Department of Forestry Pretoria.

Verghese, J. *et al.* (1987) A fresh look at the constituents of Indian Olibanum oil. *Flav. Fragr. J.* **2**, 99–102.

Wajda-Dubois, J.P. *et al.* (1996) Comparative study on the lipid fraction of pulp and seeds of *Serenoa repens* (Palmaceae). *Oleagineux Corps. Gras. Lipides.* **3**, 136–139.

Weekes, E. (1999) The incidence of malnutrition in medical patients admitted to hospital in south London. *Proc. Nutr. Soc.* **58**, 126A.

WHO (1999a) *Radix Echinacea; Herba Echinaceae Purpureae. WHO Monographs on Selected Medicinal Plants.* Vol. 1. World Health Organization, Geneva, Switzerland, pp. 125–144.

WHO (1999b) *Radix Ginkgo. WHO Monographs on Selected Medicinal Plants.* Vol. 1. World Health Organization, Geneva, Switzerland, pp. 154–167.

WHO (1999c) *Radix Ginseng. WHO Monographs on Selected Medicinal Plants.* Vol. 1. World Health Organization, Geneva, Switzerland, pp. 168–182.

WHO (2002a) Folim cum Flore Crataegi. *WHO Monographs on Selected Medicinal Plants.* Vol. 2. World Health Organization, Geneva, Switzerland, pp. 66–82.

WHO (2002b) *Cortex Pruni Africanae. WHO Monographs on Selected Medicinal Plants.* Vol. 2. World Health Organization, Geneva, Switzerland, pp. 246–258.

WHO (2009a) *Gummi Boswellii. WHO Monographs on Selected Medicinal Plants.* Vol. 4. World Health Organization, Geneva, Switzerland, pp. 48–60.

WHO (2009b) *Radix Panacis Quinquefolii. WHO Monographs on Selected Medicinal Plants.* Vol. 4. World Health Organization, Geneva, Switzerland, pp. 226–243.

WHO (2009c) *Fructus Serenoa Repentis. WHO Monographs on Selected Medicinal Plants.* Vol. 2. World Health Organization, Geneva, Switzerland, pp. 285–299.

WHO (2010) Ageing. www.who.int/topics/ageing/en/.

Wilt, T., Ishani, A., Mac Donald, R., Rutks, I. and Stark, G. (2002) *Pygeum africanum* for benign prostatic hyperplasia. *Cochrane Database Syst Rev.* (1):CD001044.

Wichtl, M. (2002) *Teedrigen und Phytopharmaka.* Wissenschaftliche Verlagsgesellschaft mbh Stuttgart.

Woelkart, K., Linde, K. and Bauer, R. (2008) Echinacea for preventing and treating the common cold. *Planta Med.* **74**, 633–637.

Wolsko, P.M., Eisenberg, D.M., Davis, R.B., Ettner, S.L. and Phillips, R.S. (2002) Insurance coverage, medical conditions, and visits to alternative medicine providers: Results of a national survey. *Arch. Intern. Med.* **162**, 281–287.

Yi, S.W., Sull, J.W., Hong, J.S., Linton, J.A. and Ohrr, H. (2009) Association between ginseng intake and mortality: Kangwha cohort study. *J Altern. Complem. Med.* **15**, 921–928.

Yuan, C.S., Wei, G., Dey, L., Karrison, T., Nahlik, L., Maleckar, S., Kasza, K., Ang-Lee, M. and Moss, J. (2004). Brief communication: American ginseng reduces warfarin's effect in healthy patients: A randomized, controlled Trial. *Ann. Intern. Med.* **141**, 23–27.

Zhang, Y., Lu, S. and Liu, Y.Y. (2007) [Effect of *Panax quinquefolius* saponin on insulin sensitivity in patients of coronary heart disease with blood glucose abnormality]. [Article in Chinese]. *Zhongguo Zhong Xi Yi Jie He Za Zhi.* **27**, 1066–1069.

Zick, S.M, Vautaw, BM, Gillespie, B. and Aaronson, K.D. (2009) Hawthorne extract randomized blinded chronic heart failure (HERB CHF) trial. *Eur. J. Heart Fail.* **11**, 990–999.

Chapter 5

Chinese Functional Foods for Aging — Individual Choices

Zhi-Xiu Lin

Abstract

Chinese herbal medicines have been used to treat age-related diseases for a long time. Some Chinese medicines are also being used as functional food items in daily cooking for health maintenance and disease prevention purposes. This article provides an overview of the theories and principles underpinning the application of Chinese functional foods for health maintenance, especially in an aged population. The pathophysiology of aging is reviewed from a Chinese medical perspective, and the decline of kidney essence, the reduction of visceral functions and the accumulation of pathogenic products such as phlegm turbidity and blood stasis are identified as the basic mechanisms that drive the aging process. Accordingly, herbs with the functions of tonifying kidney essence, strengthening the *qi* and blood, resolving phlegm and invigorating blood circulation are the main ingredients for anti-aging applications. According to China's Ministry of Health, 87 Chinese herbs can be used as edible food items. Another 113 Chinese herbs can be classified as health promotion ingredients. These two categories of herbs are collectively called Chinese functional foods. The use of these Chinese functional foods for health promotion should conform to the basic principles of Chinese medicine. A number of functional food formulas are cited as examples to illustrate the application of Chinese functional ingredients for promoting health conditions among old people.

Keywords: Chinese Medicine; Functional Foods; Aging; Anti-Aging; Health Promotion.

5.1 Introduction

The average life expectancy has dramatically increased in the past half a century, and there are currently more than 130 million elderly people (i.e. older than 60 years) in China, accounting for about 10% of its total population (Li, 2005). It is projected that by the middle of the twenty-first century the number of elderly people in China will reach 400 million (Jiang *et al.*, 2004). With the advent of an aging society, there has been a significant increase in the incidence of age-related diseases. For example, more than five million elderly people in China have been diagnosed with Alzheimer's disease (AD), representing about one quarter of the world's total patient population of this devastating disease. The situation is not going to become any easier in the foreseeable future, as on average about 300,000 new cases of AD will be reported in China each year (Jiang *et al.*, 2004). Needless to say, age-related diseases place a heavy economic burden both on the patients' families and on society as a whole. According to a survey conducted by the Beijing Elderly People's Association, the cost to an average family for taking care of a severe AD patient is about RBM 20,000 per annum. In the United States of America, the direct and indirect economic loss due to this disease is approximately US$100 billion per year; and it is estimated that the USA will save about US$500 million if the occurrence of AD can be postponed for five years.

During the past few decades, health protection and maintenance, nutritional and psychiatric support in elderly population and the treatment of geriatric conditions have become popular research areas worldwide. In China, where there exists a rich tradition and culture in life nurturing and health preservation, the practice of active promotion of healthy aging, prevention and delaying of age-related diseases, and cultivation for longevity has been given an important place in the nation's healthcare strategy. In this endeavor, Chinese medicine is often viewed and used as a time-honored tool. At the community practical level, many herbal medicines are widely incorporated into elderly people's daily diets with the explicit aims of promoting health, preventing disease and enhancing quality of life. The widespread use of Chinese medicines for food consumption is perhaps the most striking feature in healthcare for the aged in Chinese society. This paper provides an overview of the application of Chinese functional foods for the purpose of health maintenance in the aged population. Along the way, the underlying principles governing the use of Chinese functional foods, and the treatment strategies employed in the use of the medicines-as-foods will be discussed so as to provide essential background knowledge in this subject area. In addition, the pathophysiology regarding aging process and the rationale underpinning its management from Chinese medicine perspective will be reviewed. Lastly, examples of individual choices of Chinese functional foods for general health promotion and alleviation of certain common geriatric conditions will be described.

5.2 Aging from the Perspective of Chinese Medicine

According to the basic theories of Chinese medicine, kidney essence (a refined substance housed in the kidney) is intimately associated with all stages of human life including birth, growth, development, reproduction and aging. The gradual diminishing of the kidney essence and deterioration of the kidney functions are the underlying driving force for the ageing process. Correspondingly, kidney essence and functions are the fundamental factors that need to be addressed if the aging process can be delayed. As one of the visceral organs of the human body, the kidney holds an important place in the terms of development and aging, because the human essence stored in the kidney is the basic substance responsible for growth, development and reproduction. With advancing age, the kidney essence starts to decline, and the reproductive function also diminishes, as do other bodily structures and functions. As a result of this process, signs of general senescence begin to appear, such as grey hair, loosening teeth, decline of hearing and eyesight, fragility of bones, soreness of lower back and weakness of the legs, withering of muscles, and a tendency to forgetfulness. In general, the quality of life of the elderly is poorer than that of younger people.

Because the human body is an organic unity, the kidney is closely linked to other visceral organs and meridians of the body. The decline of the kidney's functions will inevitably affect other visceral organs and lead to the deficiency and malfunction of other organs such as the deficiency of the spleen and stomach *qi*, weakness of the lung *qi* and malfunction of the heart *qi*. Dysregulated visceral functions consequently reduce the body's defence ability and predispose it to the invasion of various pathogenic factors. For individuals exposed to unwanted emotional stress, dietary irregularity, and overexertion, all these negative factors will expedite the weakness of the visceral organs and break the harmony of the *qi* and blood of the body. The aberrant *qi* and blood circulation can give rise to the production of phlegm turbidity and blood stasis. In the etiology of Chinese medicine, phlegm and blood stasis are two internal pathogenic factors respectively arising from the dysfunction of water metabolism and blood circulation. It has been established that the production of phlegm and blood stasis is very common in elderly people (Yu, 1992; Yang, 2002). These endogenous pathogenic products in turn further interfere with the normal physiological production and the circulation of *qi* and blood. Moreover, the accumulation of phlegm and blood stasis causes visceral malfunction, and weakens the body's genuine *qi*. All these pathogenic mechanisms will contribute to the aging process.

From the perspective of Chinese medicine, common age-related diseases such as chronic obstructive pulmonary disease (COPD), coronary heart disease, atherosclerosis, hypertension, stroke, Alzheimer's disease, vascular dementia and cancers are the direct results of disharmony of visceral functions and the accumulation of pathogenic products such as phlegm and blood stasis. Taken together, Chinese medicine regards aging as a slow and chronic process involving the temporal decline of visceral functions, particularly that of the kidney, together with the inevitable production and accumulation of phlegm and blood stasis in the meridians and visceral organs. Therefore, to help slow down the aging process, it is necessary to address the kidney deficiency and resolve the accumulation of phlegm and blood stagnation. Indeed, many anti-aging Chinese functional foods hold out the promise of tonifying the kidney essence, strengthening the kidney *qi*, resolving phlegm and invigorating blood circulation and removing blood stasis (Lu, 2001).

5.3 Chinese Medicines Used as Functional Foods

The past few decades have witnessed an upsurge of interest around the world in the consumption of functional foods for health maintenance and disease prevention. The term "functional" food was first used in Japan in the 1960s, and similar terms are now used in other countries to refer to foods of this nature. For example, in Germany functional foods are called "improvement foods", while "therapeutic foods" are commonly used in Korea, and "dietary supplements" in the USA (Dang *et al.*, 1999).

Functional food is any fresh or processed food that has a health-promoting and/or disease-preventing property beyond the basic nutritional function of supplying nutrients. In other words, any dietary item containing components that provide additional health benefits on top of the nutrients necessary for normal metabolic activity can be regarded as a functional food. According to the US Dietary Supplement Health and Education Act of 1994, a dietary supplement is defined as a substance that is intended to supplement the diet, contains one or more dietary ingredients (including vitamins, minerals, herbs or other botanicals, amino acids, and other substances) or their constituents, is intended to be taken by mouth as a pill, capsule, tablet or liquid, and is labeled on the front panel as being a dietary supplement.

In China, Chinese herbal medicines have been used for the treatment of various diseases as well as health maintenance and wellness promotion since time immemorial. The use of medicinal herbs has always been an important component in Chinese culture. The *Shen Nong Ben Cao Jing* (Divine Husbandman's Materia Medica), the first specialist book on Chinese herbal medicine, written about 2000 years ago, documents the use of 365 herbs and details their functions and indications. These 365 medicinal substances are broadly categorized into three classes according to their therapeutic functions, *viz.* top-grade, medium-grade and low-grade medicinals. The top-grade medicinals are those that are non-toxic and can be consumed for long periods of time without harmful side effects. Some herbs in this category, such as *Ginseng radix* (*Ren shen*), *Astragalus radix* (*Huang qi*), *Dioscoreae rhizoma* (*Shan yao*), *Angelica sinensis radix* (*Dang gui*) and *Jujubae fructus* (*Da zao*), are still being used as functional foods for health maintenance and disease prevention today. The medium-grade herbs are those that are non-toxic or are slightly toxic, and can be used to treat disease and to supplement vital *qi* deficiency. Low-grade medicinals refer to the substances that are toxic or harsh in their actions, which cannot be taken for long periods of time, and are mainly used to remove heat and cold evil and to resolve pathogenic accumulations.

Over the centuries, the number of medicinal herbs used in Chinese medicine practice has increased steadily, and by the middle of the last century, the number of materia medica commonly employed in Chinese medicine had reached about 5700 (Jiangsu New Medical College, 1985). Some of the many herbs used in Chinese medicine can not only be prescribed for the treatment of diseases but can also be used as edible food items owing to their tonifying nature, mildness in action, and lack of side effects. Table 1 lists 87 herbs in this category that have been specifically endorsed by the Ministry of Health (2002a) as having dual roles as medicines and foods. Another 113 Chinese herbs have also been classified as herbs with a health promotion capability, although they are not generally categorized as food items (Ministry of Health, 2002b). In the broad context, both of these two groups of herbs can be regarded as Chinese functional foods because their consumption can elicit health promotion effects, and they are nowadays commonly incorporated into daily diets and culinary practice in various forms, such as soup, decoction, congee, juice, tincture, paste, jelly and candy for the purpose of preservation and promotion of good health, and relieving symptoms of diseases. This practice echoes a Chinese saying "Medicine and food share the same origin", implying that certain Chinese medicines can be consumed as foods, and vice versa. Since some of these herbs are alleged to possess an anti-aging effect, they are often used as functional foods for promoting the general well-being of elderly people.

5.4 Principles of Using Chinese Functional Foods for Health Promotion

Western nutritional theory emphasizes the macro- and micro-nutritional contents of particular food items, such as protein, fat, sugar, minerals, vitamins and fibre. By contrast Chinese functional foods are used in accordance with ancient medical theories that govern the practice of Chinese herbal medicine, in particular classification into four natures (cold, cool, hot and warm) and five tastes (acrid (pungent), sweet, bitter, sour and salty), and a focus on the channels entering and sites of action. The four natures refers to the temperature characteristics regarding the response of the human body to the influence of a given herb, and they are termed as cold, hot,

Table 5.1. List of Chinese herbal medicines which are suitable for food consumption.

Chinese name	Pharmaceutical name	Properties	Channel(s) entered	Key characteristic(s)
丁香	*Caryophylli Flos*	Acrid, warm	Kidney, spleen, stomach	Warms the middle, directs stomach *qi* downward, treats hiccough, fortifies the kidney *yang*.
八角茴香	*Illicii Fructus*	Acrid, warm	Liver, kidney, spleen, stomach	Harmonizes the middle, warms the lower burner, treats bulging disorders.
刀豆	*Canavaliae Semen*	Sweet, warm	Spleen, kidney	Drives *qi* downward to stop hiccough, warms and tonifies the kidney.
小茴香	*Foeniculi Fructus*	Acrid, warm	Liver, kidney, spleen, stomach	Harmonizes the middle, warms the lower burner, treats bulging disorders.
小薊	*Cirsii Herba*	Sweet, cool	Liver, heart	Cools the blood and stops bleeding, promotes urination.
山藥	*Dioscoreae Rhizoma*	Sweet, neutral	Kidney, lung, spleen	Tonifies the *qi* and *yin* of the lung, spleen, and kidney; secures the essence.
山楂	*Crataegi Fructus*	Sour, sweet, slightly warm	Liver, spleen, stomach	Relieves food stagnation, especially from meat and greasy foods, invigorates the blood circulation, alleviates diarrhea and dysentery.
馬 莧	*Portulacae Herba*	Sour, cold, slippery	Large intestine, liver	Clears heat and resolves toxicity, eases the intestines.
烏梢蛇	*Zaocys*	Sweet, salty, neutral	Liver, spleen	Dispels wind, unblocks the collaterals, stops convulsions.
烏梅	*Mume Fructus*	Sour, astringent, warm	Large intestine, liver, lung, spleen	Preserves the lung, binds up the intestine, stops bleeding, generates fluids, quiets intestinal parasites.

(Continued)

Table 5.1. (*Continued*)

Chinese name	Pharmaceutical name	Properties	Channel(s) entered	Key characteristic(s)
木瓜	*Chaenomelis Fructus*	Sour, warm	Liver, spleen	Transforms dampness, harmonizes the spleen and stomach, alleviates cramping.
火麻仁	*Cannabis Semen*	Sweet, neutral	Large intestine, spleen, stomach	Enriches the *yin* fluids, moistens the intestines, unblocks dry constipation.
代代花	*Aurantii Fructus (unripe)*	Bitter, acrid, slightly cold	Spleen, stomach, large intestine	Promotes the flow of *qi*, unblocks plugs.
玉竹	*Polygonati odorati Rhizoma*	Sweet, slightly cold	Lung, stomach	Enriches the lung and stomach *yin*, restores body fluids.
甘草	*Glycyrrhizae Radix*	Sweet, neutral (unprepared); sweet, warm (dry-fried)	All 12 channels, especially the heart, lung, spleen and stomach	Tonifies the spleen *qi*, moistens the lung, moderates urgency and toxicity, drains fire.
白芷	*Angelicae dahuricae Radix*	Acrid, warm	Lung, stomach, spleen	Releases the exterior, opens the orifices (especially the nose), dries dampness.
白果	*Ginkgo Semen*	Sweet, bitter, astringent, neutral, slightly toxic	Kidney, lung	Treats phlegm-heat cough and wheezing, eliminates turbid damp vaginal discharge.

(*Continued*)

Table 5.1. (*Continued*)

Chinese name	Pharmaceutical name	Properties	Channel(s) entered	Key characteristic(s)
白扁豆	*Dolichos Semen*	Sweet, slightly warm	Spleen, stomach	Strengthens the spleen, transforms dampness and clears summerheat.
白扁豆花	*Dolichos Flos*	Sweet, bland, neutral	Spleen, stomach	Clears summerheat, transforms dampness.
眼肉 (桂圓)	*Longan Arillus*	Sweet, warm	Heart, spleen	Nourishes the blood, tonifies the *qi*, calms the spirit.
決明子	*Cassiae Semen*	Bitter, sweet, salty, slightly cold	Liver, large intestine, kidney	Disperses wind-fire to cool the eyes, moistens the intestines, nourishes the liver and kidney *yin*.
百合	*Lilii Bulbus*	Sweet, slightly bitter, slightly cold	Heart, lung	Enriches the lung *yin*, drains the heart heat, stops coughs, tranquilises the spirit.
肉豆蔻	*Myristicae Semen*	Acrid, warm	Large intestine, spleen, stomach	Warms the spleen and stomach, promotes the movement of *qi*, binds up the intestines.
肉桂	*Cinnamomi Cortex*	Acrid, sweet, hot	Heart, kidney, liver, spleen	Warms and tonifies the yang, disperses cold, promotes the movement of blood.
余甘子	*Phyllanti Fructus*	Sweet, sour, astringent, cool	Lung, stomach	Clears the lung to benefit the throat, transforms phlegm to stop cough, generates body fluids.
佛手	*Citri sarcodactylis Fructus*	Acrid, bitter, warm	Liver, lung, stomach, spleen	Regulates the *qi*, relieves constraint, transforms phlegm, harmonizes the middle.

(*Continued*)

Table 5.1. (*Continued*)

Chinese name	Pharmaceutical name	Properties	Channel(s) entered	Key characteristic(s)
杏仁 (甜、苦)	*Armeniacae Semen*	Bitter, slightly warm, slightly toxic	Lung, large intestine	Directs the lung *qi* downward, disperses wind-cold, moistens the intestines.
沙棘	*Hippophae Fructus*	Sour, astringent, slightly sweet, warm	Lung, spleen, stomach, large intestine	Augments the *qi*, generates fluids, stops coughs, assists digestion.
牡蠣	*Ostreae Concha*	Salty, astringent, cool	Liver, kidney	Secures deficiency leading to leakage and loss; softens masses or nodules due to constrained heat and phlegm.
芡實	*Euryales Semen*	Sweet, astringent, neutral	Kidney, spleen	Tonifies and restrains the spleen and kidney, eliminates dampness.
花椒	*Zanthoxyli Pericarpium*	Acrid, hot, slightly toxic	Kidney, spleen, stomach	Warms the middle, disperses cold, stops pain, kills parasites, tonifies fire at the gate of vitality.
赤小豆	*Phaseoli Semen*	Sweet, sour, neutral	Heart, small intestine	Treats both damp edema and toxic fire.
阿膠	*Asini Corii Colla*	Sweet, neutral	Kidney, liver, lung	Tonifies liver blood, moistens lung *yin*, replenishes kidney essence, stops bleeding.
雞內金	*Gigeriae galli Endothelium corneum*	Sweet, neutral	Bladder, small intestine, spleen	Reduces all types of food stagnation, stops enuresis, dissolves stones.
麥芽	*Hordei Fructus germinatus*	Sweet, neutral	Liver, spleen, stomach	Reduces food stagnation due to starches and fruits, improves the appetite.

(*Continued*)

Table 5.1. (*Continued*)

Chinese name	Pharmaceutical name	Properties	Channel(s) entered	Key characteristic(s)
昆布	*Eckloniae Thallus*	Salty, cold	Kidney, liver, stomach	Reduces phlegm and softens areas of hardness, promotes urination, eliminates edema.
棗（大棗、酸棗、黑棗）	*Jujubae Fructus*	Sweet, warm	Spleen, stomach	Tonifies the *qi* and blood, generates fluids, harmonizes the spleen, moderates the toxic effects of other herbs.
羅漢果	*Momordicae Fructus*	Sweet, cool	Lung, large intestine	Clears heat and moistens the lung, generates fluids to stop thirst, lubricates the intestines to open the bowels.
郁李仁	*Pruni Semen*	Acrid, bitter, sweet, neutral	Large and small intestines, spleen	Moistens and drains downward; treats constipation and the retention of fluids.
金銀花	*Lonicerae Flos*	Sweet, cold	Large intestine, lung, stomach	Disperses heat, resolves toxicity, cools the blood.
青果	*Canarii Fructus*	Sweet, sour, neutral	Lung, stomach, spleen	Generates fluids, benefits the throat, resolves alcoholic intoxication.
魚腥草	*Houttuyniae Herba*	Acrid, cool	Lung, large intestine	Disperses heat, resolves toxicity, reduces swelling, acts especially on the lung.
薑（生薑、乾薑）	*Zingiberis Rhizoma*	Acrid, slightly warm	Lung, spleen, stomach	Benefits the stomach, alleviates nausea, stops coughing, transforms phlegm.
枳椇子	*Hovenia Fructus*	Sweet, sour, neutral	Heart, spleen	Clears heat, relieves thirst.

(*Continued*)

Table 5.1. (*Continued*)

Chinese name	Pharmaceutical name	Properties	Channel(s) entered	Key characteristic(s)
枸杞子	*Lycii Fructus*	Sweet, neutral	Liver, lung, kidney	Enriches the *yin* of the kidney and lung, nourishes the liver blood, mildly tonifies the kidney *yang*.
栀子	*Gardeniae Fructus*	Bitter, cold	Heart, lung, stomach, liver, triple burner	Resolves constrained heat, dries dampness, cools the blood, breaks up toxic accumulations.
砂仁	*Amomi Fructus*	Acrid, warm, aromatic	Spleen, stomach	Promotes the flow of *qi*, warms the middle, transforms dampness, improves the appetite, calms the fetus.
胖大海	*Sterculiae lychnophorae Semen*	Sweet, cold	Large intestine, lung	Gently cools and moistens the throat and intestines.
茯苓	*Poria*	Sweet, bland, neutral	Heart, spleen, kidney, lung	Tonifies the spleen, eliminates dampness, calms the heart spirit.
香橼	*Citri Fructus*	Acrid, slightly bitter, sour, warm	Liver, spleen, lung	Transforms phlegm to stop coughs, regulates the *qi* and relieves constraint to alleviate epigastric pain, stops nausea, improves appetite.
香薷	*Moslae Herba*	Acrid, aromatic, slightly warm	Lung, stomach	Assists the *yang qi* to expel pathogenic wind, harmonizes the spleen and transforms dampness.
桃仁	*Persicae Semen*	Bitter, sweet, neutral	Heart, large intestine, liver, lung,	Invigorates the blood, removes stasis, moistens the intestines, stops coughs and wheezing.
桑叶	*Mori Folium*	Sweet, bitter, cold	Lung, liver	Disperses wind-heat, cools and drains the lung and liver.
桑椹	*Mori Fructus*	Sweet, cold	Heart, liver, kidney	Gently nourishes and cools the blood and *yin*.

(*Continued*)

Table 5.1. (*Continued*)

Chinese name	Pharmaceutical name	Properties	Channel(s) entered	Key characteristic(s)
桔红	*Citri reticulatae Exocarpium rubrum*	Acrid, bitter, warm	Lung, stomach	Dries phlegm-dampness to stop coughs.
桔梗	*Platycodi Radix*	Bitter, acrid, neutral	Lung	Soothes the throat, releases the exterior, transforms phlegm, expels pus.
益智仁	*Alpiniae oxyphyllae Fructus*	Acrid, warm	Kidney, spleen	Warmly tonifies the spleen and kidney *yang*, secures the urine.
荷葉	*Nelumbinis Folium*	Bitter, slightly sweet, neutral	Heart, liver, spleen	Clears heat, resolves summerheat, raises clear *yang*, stops bleeding.
莱菔子	*Raphani Semen*	Acrid, sweet, neutral	Lung, spleen, stomach	Transforms phlegm, reduces food stagnation, promotes the flow of *qi* in the lung, spleen and large intestine.
蓮子	*Nelumbinis Semen*	Sweet, astringent, neutral	Heart, kidney, spleen	Tonifies and stabilizes the spleen, heart, and kidney, calms the spirit.
高良薑	*Alpiniae officinarum Rhizoma*	Acrid, hot	Spleen, stomach	Warms the stomach, disperses cold, stops pain, directs rebellious *qi* downward.
淡竹葉	*Lophateri Herba*	Sweet, bland, cold	Heart, small intestine, stomach	Drains dampness and promotes urination, relieves irritability associated with heat.

(*Continued*)

Table 5.1. (*Continued*)

Chinese name	Pharmaceutical name	Properties	Channel(s) entered	Key characteristic(s)
淡豆豉	*Sojae Semen preparatum*	Sweet, slightly bitter, cold or warm depending on the method of preparation.	Lung, stomach	Vents and expels exterior pathogens, disseminates and disperses constrained heat above the diaphragm.
菊花	*Chrysanthemi Flos*	Sweet, bitter, slightly cold	Lung, liver	Disperses wind-heat, cools and tonifies the liver and brightens the eyes and resolves toxicity.
菊苣	*Cichorii Herba*	Bitter, cold,	Liver, gallbladder	Clears liver heat and benefits gallbladder.
黄芥子	*Sinapis Semen*	Acrid, warm	lung	Transforms cold-phlegm, dissipates clumps.
黄精	*Polygonati Rhizoma*	Sweet, neutral	Kidney, lung, spleen	Tonifies the *qi*, nourishes the *yin*, augments the essence.
紫蘇	*Perillae Folium*	Acrid, aromatic, warm	Lung, spleen	Harmonizes the middle, promotes *qi* movement and revives the spleen.
紫蘇籽	*Perillae Fructus*	Acrid, warm	Large intestine, lung	Directs *qi* downward to disperse phlegm and calm wheezing, moistens the intestines.
葛根	*Puerariae Radix*	Sweet, acrid, cool	Spleen, stomach	Raises the clear *yang qi*, releases muscle layer heat and vents rashes, alleviates thirst by raising stomach fluids, treats diarrhea.
黑芝麻	*Sesami Semen nigrum*	Sweet, neutral	Kidney, liver, large intestine	Tonifies the liver and kidney, augments the *yin* and blood, lubricates the intestines.
黑胡椒	*Piperis Fructus*	Acrid, hot	Large intestine, stomach	Eliminates pathogenic cold in the stomach and intestines.

(*Continued*)

Table 5.1. (*Continued*)

Chinese name	Pharmaceutical name	Properties	Channel(s) entered	Key characteristic(s)
槐米	*Sophorae Flos immaturus*	Bitter, cold	Liver, large intestine	Cools the blood, clears heat, stops bleeding.
槐花	*Sophora Flos*	Bitter, cold	Liver, large intestine	Cools the blood, clears heat, stops bleeding.
蒲公英	*Taraxaci Herba*	Bitter, sweet, cold	Liver, stomach	Cools heat, resolves toxicity, directs downward, facilitates urination.
蜂蜜	*Honey*	Sweet, neutral	Lung, spleen, large intestine	Tonifies the middle to alleviate pain, moistens and resolves toxicity.
榧子	*Torreyae Semen*	Sweet, neutral	Large intestine, lung, stomach	Kills parasites without injuring the spleen and stomach, moistens the lung and stops coughs.
酸枣仁	*Ziziphi spinosae Semen*	Sweet, sour neutral	Gallbladder, heart, liver, spleen	Nourishes the heart *yin* and liver blood, promotes sleep, inhibits sweating.
鮮白茅根	*Imperatae Rhizoma (fresh)*	Sweet, cold	Lung, stomach, small intestine	Cools the blood, stops bleeding, clears heat in the lung and stomach, promotes urination.
鮮蘆根	*Phragmitis Rhizoma (fresh)*	Sweet, cold	Lung, stomach	Cools the lung and stomach, generates fluids, alleviates nausea, promotes urination.
蝮蛇	*Agkistrodon*	Sweet, warm, toxic (venom)	Liver	Quenches wind to stop spasm.

(*Continued*)

Table 5.1. (*Continued*)

Chinese name	Pharmaceutical name	Properties	Channel(s) entered	Key characteristic(s)
橘皮	*Citri reticulatae Pericarpium*	Acrid, bitter, warm, aromatic	Lung, spleen, stomach	Promotes the flow of *qi*, dries dampness.
薄荷	*Menthae haplocalycis Herba*	Acrid, aromatic, cool	Lung, liver	Clears wind-heat, cools and clears the eyes and head, soothes the throat, facilitates the flow of liver *qi* and expels turbid filth.
薏苡仁	*Coicis Semen*	Sweet, bland, slightly cold	Lung, spleen, stomach, kidney	Tonifies the spleen and augments the lung, expels dampness, cools heat and expels pus to treat sores and abscesses.
薤白	*Allii macrostemi Bulbus*	Acrid, bitter, warm	Large intestine, lung, stomach	Reaches into areas of congealed constraint to unblock and benefit the orifices.
覆盆子	*Rubi Fructus*	Sweet, astringent, neutral	Kidney, liver	Augments the kidney *yin*, contains the urine, secures the essence.
藿香	*Pogostemonis Herba*	Acrid, slightly warm	Lung, spleen, stomach	Releases the exterior, transforms dampness, harmonizes the middle, alleviates nausea.

warm and cool. The cold and cool natures belong to the same character, and they only vary in degree of coldness (cold is more severe than cool). Similarly, the hot and warm natures belong to the same character, and they only vary in severity of hotness (hot is more severe than warm). If a herb is neither hot or cold, or the hotness and coldness of the herb is not obvious, it is usually called neutral. In terms of the action of herbs, herbs with cold or cool nature normally have the effects of heat-clearing, fire-purging, detoxification and *yin*-nourishing, and are mainly used for the treatment of heat syndromes. Conversely, herbs with a hot or warm nature normally have the functions of cold-dispersing, interior-warming, *yang*-enhancing, and collapse-reversing, and are generally used for cold syndromes.

The five flavors is another basic theory of Chinese materia medica. The five flavors refers to the five basic sensory perceptions that describe the flavors of herbs when ingested. These flavors are, respectively, acrid (also called pungent), sweet, sour, bitter and salty. However, some herbs may have a bland or astringent taste. The flavors dictate the effects and actions. Thus, herbs that have different tastes usually have dissimilar pharmacological effects and therapeutic actions, while herbs with similar tastes usually have similar effects and actions. The flavor-action relationships are largely based on empirical experience of the long history of Chinese medicine practice. Table 2 shows the flavors of herbs and their respective functions and indications.

The theory of herbs entering specific channels refers to a herb's selective therapeutic effects on specific parts of the body, including channels and organs. According to this theory, a herb may exert obvious therapeutic actions on one or several specific channels or viscera, while having little or no effects on other channels or organs. Throughout the long history of herbal medicine practice, experience has been accumulated in establishing the channels entered by various herbs. For example, *Armeniacae Semen (Xing ren)* is effective for cough, asthma, and pain in the chest, so it is ascribed to the lung channel. Because *Xing ren* is able to lubricate the large intestine to relieve constipation, it also enters the large intestine channel.

By taking together the theories of four natures, five flavors and channel entering, it is possible to know the nature (hotness or coldness) and inclination of the herb in respect of specific organs, and to define the herb's therapeutic functions and clinical indications.

Table 5.2. Effects and indications of herbs with different flavors.

Flavor	Functions and indications	Examples of herbs
Acrid (pungent)	Dispersing exopathogens from the skin; promoting the circulation of *qi* and blood.	*Piperis Fructus; Zanthoxyli Pericarpium; Zingiberis Rhizoma*
Sweet	Nourishing and tonifying the body; harmonizing the functions of spleen and stomach; harmonizing different herbs in a formula, and alleviating spasm and pain.	*Jujubae Fructus;* Honey; *Glycyrrhizae Radix*
Sour	Inducing astringency and arresting discharge. Herbs of sour flavor are used to treat excessive sweating due to deficiency, chronic cough, usually without much phlegm, chronic diarrhea, emission, spermatorrhea, enuresis, and various bleeding.	*Hippophae Fructus; Canarii Fructus*
Astringent	Has similar effects as the sour flavor; can be used to treat emission, and chronic diarrhea.	*Nelumbinis Semen; Rubi Fructus*
Bitter	Clearing heat and purging fire; sending down the adverse flow of *qi* to treat cough and vomiting; purging the bowels, and eliminating dampness.	*Armeniacae Semen; Cichorii Herba*
Salty	Softening and resolving the hard masses, and opening the bowels by purgation.	*Ostreae Concha; Eckloniae Thallus*
Bland	Excreting dampness and inducing diuresis. Herbs of bland flavor are used to treat edema and dysuria (difficulty in passing water).	*Coicis Semen; Lophateri Herba*

The basic concept in Chinese medicine is that a healthy body is the result of a balance of *yin* and *yang*; and that the disturbance of this balance leads to disease. Several fundamental strategies are used in Chinese medicine practice to guide the selection of herbs for treatment of disease. These are: (1) heat-type condition (symptoms may include fever, red complexion, sweating, thirst, irritability, constipation, scant and deep colour urine, yellow tongue coating and rapid pulse) should be treated with drug of cool/cold nature. (2) Cold condition (symptoms may include aversion to cold, cold extremities, abdominal or lower back pain and weakness of the knees, frequent urination at night, pale tongue with white coating, slow pulse) should be treated with drugs of warm/hot nature. (3) Using reducing methods to relieve excesses in order to restore balance. Excesses are caused by invasion of pathogenic factors such as wind, cold, damp, heat, summerheat, dryness, phlegm and blood stasis. (4) Using nourishing and reinforcing method to treat deficiency and vacuity. In Chinese medicine, any insufficiency in the body's *qi*, blood, *yin* and *yang* is called a deficient condition.

These principles are duly applied to Chinese functional foods. Food recipes containing these Chinese functional ingredients can be designed specifically for elderly people. Tailor-made recipes may be formulated based on an elderly person's body constitution, health condition and the nature of disease. The climate and geographical locations should also be considered when formulating food recipes. The incorporation of Chinese functional foods in daily diet is expected to strengthen the constitution of elderly people and improve their defence function so as to prevent the occurrence of disease, and to complement medical treatment.

5.5 Chinese Functional Foods for Aging

As discussed above, aging as a physiological and pathogenic process is closely associated with the deficiency of kidney essence and *qi*, together with deterioration of the physiological functions of other organs such as the spleen, the heart and the lung. In addition, the endogenous pathogenic products such as phlegm turbidity and blood stasis are also important etiological factors for age-related diseases. Therefore, the Chinese functional foods with the properties of: (1) tonifying the kidney function; (2) supplementing spleen and lung *qi*; (3) regulating liver *qi* and soothing stagnation; (4) dissolving phlegm; and (5) removing blood stasis, are extensively used for anti-aging purpose.

During the past few decades, many studies have attempted to elucidate the anti-aging mechanisms of some Chinese herbs. The publications in this area are voluminous. A comprehensive coverage of anti-aging herbs is beyond the scope of this article, and only a few examples are cited here to illustrate what has been discovered about the anti-aging properties of some common Chinese functional food ingredients together with their action mechanisms.

Fructus Lycii (Gou qi zi) is a widely used anti-aging Chinese functional food because of its liver and kidney nourishing properties and ability to improve vision. In addition, its agreeably bright color and pleasant taste make it an attractive food item. Recent laboratory studies have demonstrated that feeding D-galactose-induced aging mice with crude polysaccharides derived from *Fructus Lycii* daily resulted in: (1) a decrease in serum advanced glycation-end products level; (2) restoration of motor activity; (3) an improvement in the memory index for animals; and (4) an increase in superoxide dismutase (SOD) levels in erythrocytes (Deng *et al.*, 2003). In another study, administration of polysaccharides from *L. barbarum* (LBP) (16 mg/kg) significantly reduced age-related oxidative stress in aged mice (Li, 2007). It has been demonstrated in a *Drosophila melanogaster* (fruit-fly) model that administration of LBP at 16 mg/kg markedly augmented the maximal and average lifespan of the male fruit-fly (Wang *et al.*, 2002). In a study involving human subjects, supplementation of diet with *Fructus Lycii* for a total of 500 mg in ten days resulted in a significant reduction in plasma triglyceride levels and an increase in plasma cAMP and SOD levels, suggesting a beneficial role of *Fructus Lycii* in human health. *Fructus Lycii* has also been shown to have an anti-diabetic effect (Luo *et al.*, 2004). Furthermore, polysaccharide fraction of *Fructus Lycii* exhibited effective prevention against chemically induced neuronal death on primary cultured neurons (Yu *et al.*, 2005; 2007). All these animal and human studies show that *Fructus Lycii* as a Chinese functional food confers its health benefits by reducing various risk factors in age-related conditions.

Rhodiola Radix (Hong jing tian). This is another Chinese functional food reputed for its promising anti-aging activity. It was shown in a recent study (Jafari *et al.*, 2007) that supplementation of *Rhodiola Radix* extract at 30 mg/ml every other day significantly increased the lifespan of *Drosophila melanogaster*. A comparison of the distribution of deaths between *Rhodiola*-supplemented and control flies demonstrated that aging was decelerated in *Rhodiola*-fed flies, indicating that *Rhodiola* is an agent that has anti-aging effects.

Ginseng Radix (*Ren shen*). Ginseng has long been regarded in Asia as the "heal-all" medicine, and is perhaps the most common oriental herb consumed for anti-aging purposes in Eastern societies such as China, Korea, Singapore and Japan. Ginseng as a renowned anti-aging natural agent, together with its many chemical constituents, has been subjected to intensive animal and clinical investigations, and the evidence for its anti-aging potential has gradually accumulated over the past few decades.

Shen *et al.* (2004) investigated the influence of ginsenoside Rg1, an active ingredient of ginseng, on the proliferation ability of rodent hippocampal progenitor cells both *in vitro* and *in vivo*. Incubation of neural progenitor cells with ginsenoside Rg1 resulted in a significant increase in the proliferation of this cell type. Furthermore, the administration of Rg1 via i.p. for two weeks caused a marked enhancement of the number of dividing cells in the hippocampus of adult mice. These findings provide evidence that the ginseng component could enhance neural cell function and possess anti-aging potential.

In another study, Nishijo *et al.* (2004) demonstrated that treatment with red ginseng significantly ameliorated place-navigation deficits in young rats with hippocampal lesion in the place learning task (PLT). Red ginseng also improved the performance of aged rats in the PLT. These observations suggested that red ginseng could enhance learning and memory deficits through effects on the central nervous system via actions on hippocampal formation.

Memory decline or total loss is a common clinical feature in aging people. Ginseng has long been used in Chinese medicine to treat memory deficiency, but the mechanism of action remains unclear. In a recent study (Zhao *et al.*, 2009), senescence-accelerated mice (SAM) were chronically treated with ginsenoside at doses of 100–200 mg/kg/day for seven consecutive months. At the end of the treatment, the β-amyloid level in the hippocampus of the SAM was markedly decreased, while the antioxidase level significantly increased in serum. In addition, plasticity-related proteins in the hippocampus were also significantly accentuated in the ginsenoside-treated groups. The findings provide experimental evidence to suggest that an increase of antioxidant and up-regulation of plasticity-related proteins in hippocampus may be the mechanisms of ginsenoside on the prevention of memory loss in aged mice.

McElhaney *et al.* (2004) conducted a randomized control trial to compare a proprietary extract of American ginseng with a placebo in preventing acute respiratory illness (ARI) in an institutional setting during the influenza season. Oral twice-daily administration of American ginseng extract 200mg resulted in a significant reduction in the occurrence of laboratory-confirmed influenza illness (LCII) ($p = 0.033$). The combined data for LCII and respiratory syncytial virus (RSV) illness were also greater in the placebo group than in the American ginseng group ($p = 0.009$). It was concluded that American ginseng was safe, well tolerated, and potentially effective for preventing ARI due to influenza and RSV.

Astragalus Radix (Huang qi). Astragalus is one of the most widely used *qi* supplementing herbs with wide application in Chinese medicine, and is often used as a dietary supplement ingredient in aging persons. The anti-aging property of Astragalus and some of its active ingredients has been the subject of both animal and clinical investigations in recent years. Astragaloside (AST) and astragalus saponin I (ASI) have been found to improve the memory of the hydrocortisone (HC)-induced senescent rats based on Y maze test. At the biochemical level, AST and ASI attenuated the [Ca2$^+$] and suppressed apoptosis of thymocytes and hippocampal neurons induced by dexamethasone. The authors concluded that AST and ASI could delay aging in HC-treated rats (Li *et al.*, 2009). In another similar study (Lei *et al.*, 2003), AST at 40 mg/kg/day, ig for ten weeks was found to ameliorate age-related alternation in both motor response (rotating rod test) and memory (step-down type passive avoidance test), and enhance the deteriorated cellular immunity in D-galactose-treated mice. It was concluded that AST has an anti-aging effect on D-gal-induced senescent mice by delaying senility of the middle-aged mice based on its ability to improve the brain function and immunomodulatory effects. In a randomized control clinical study Zhang *et al.* (2005) investigated the effect of Astragalus injection (AI) on plasma levels of apoptosis-related factors in aged patients with chronic heart failure (CHF). The results derived from the study indicated that after four weeks' treatment, the New York Heart Association grading in AI group was significantly better than that of conventional treatment group ($p < 0.05$). In addition, in AI group the left ventricular end-systolic volume (LVESV) and left ventricular end-diastolic volume (LVEDV) markedly decreased while the left ventricular ejection fraction (LVEF) increased. In comparison with the control group, sFas, sFasL, TNF-alpha and IL-6 in the AI group were significantly attenuated.

It was concluded that AI could offer benefits in improving cardiac function in the aged patients with CHF.

In an animal experiment to evaluate the protective effect of *Astragulus mongholicus* (AM) on neuronal cell apoptosis, it was revealed that AM was able to significantly inhibit neuronal apoptosis in ageing mice brains through augmenting the activity of Mn-SOD, up-regulating the expression of bcl-2 and reducing the concentration of MDA (Wei *et al.*, 2006). Interestingly, *Astragulus mongholicus* is one of the plant species used for Chinese herb *Huang qi*, an important *qi* tonifying agent in Chinese medicine and a commonly used Chinese functional food.

5.6 Examples of Using Chinese Functional Foods for Aging — Individual Choices

Chinese functional foods are usually incorporated into people's daily cooking. The addition of these functional foods to the more ordinary food items aims to add health promoting functionality to our eating. In this connection, Chinese medical theory as described above should be used to guide the selection of the appropriate herbs for a better health promotion effect. When designing a Chinese functional food recipe, it is necessary to take into consideration a person's constitution, health or disease condition, and the season and the climate. In the long history of the utilization of Chinese functional foods, many useful and effective formulas have been developed, and these formulas can be adopted and modified to suit individuals with different body constitutions and health status. As people become better educated about the importance of functional foods for their health, many specialist books on Chinese functional food recipes have been eagerly read by general readers. The following food recipes incorporating Chinese functional food ingredients with ordinary foods serve as examples of how Chinese functional foods can be used for the purpose of improving the health of elderly individuals.

(1) *Cordyceps* Duck Broth

Ingredients:

Cordyceps ten pieces, 1/2 duck (about 0.8 kg, cleaned and with internal organs removed, cut into 5 cm pieces), ginger five slices, dry tangerine peel 3 g, cooking wine 15 ml, 1/4 tsp salt.

Preparation method:
Put all the ingredients into a porcelain cooking pot and add about 2 L water. Bring the contents to boil and then simmer for 2 hrs. Eat the duck and drink the soup. The amount is good for four servings. The recipe can be used once per week for 2–3 months.

Health benefits:
Benefits the kidney and strengthens *yang*, tonifies the lung to pacify asthma, stops bleeding and transforms phlegm. It is suitable for elderly people with sexual impotence and low back pain due to kidney *yang* deficiency. People with chronic cough or asthma and general weak constitution after illness can also use this formula.

(2) *Cassiae Semen* Congee

Ingredients: Cassiae Semen (Jue ming zi) 10 g, rice 50 g, rock sugar 15 g.

Preparation method: Fry *Cassiae Semen* in a cooking wok till it becomes slightly aromatic. When it cools down, crush the fried *Cassiae Semen* to pieces, then boil it with water (about 2 L) for 30 mins to make water extract. Follow by adding the rice to the *Cassiae Semen* extract and cook for a further 1 hr to make rice congee. Finally add rock sugar to the congee and boil for additional 15 mins.

Health benefits:
The *Cassiae Semen* Congee has the function of clearing liver heat and brightening vision, and moistening the intestines to open the bowels. It is suitable for elderly persons who are hypertensive, hyperlipidemic, obese or have habitual constipation.

(3) Herbal Congee for Insomnia

Ingredients: Ziziphi spinosae Semen (Suan zao yen) (fried) 10 g, *Nelumbinis Semen (Lian zi)* 30 g, *Longan Arillus (Long yan rou)* 15 g, rice 50 g.

Preparation method: Crush the fried *Ziziphi spinosae Semen* to pieces, then boil it in water (about 2 L) for 30 mins to make its water extract. Then put the rest of the ingredients and the *Ziziphi semen* water extract into a porcelain cooking pot and boil them further for about 1.5 hr until the rice becomes soft and loose congee. Serve the congee two or three times a day. The formula can be used twice weekly for one to two months.

Health benefits: This congee recipe has the function of strengthening the spleen and calming the mind to promote sleep. It is suitable for elderly people with insomnia and forgetfulness.

(4) *Ginkgo Folium* **and** *Crataegi Fructus* **Tea**

Ingredients: Chrysanthemi Flos (*Juhua*) 6 g, *Ginkgo Folium* (*Yin xing ye*) 6 g, *Crataegi Fructus* (*Shan zha*) 6 g, *Paeoniae Radix* (*Bai shao*) 9 g.

Preparation method: Brew the ingredients in boiling water to make water extract, which can be served as ordinary tea. The above dosage is for one day.

Health benefits:
This tea formula is used for dementia associated with hypertension and atherosclerosis.

5.7 Discussion

Chinese herbal medicines have long been used as functional foods to nurture life, to preserve and enhance health, to prevent disease and to supplement various treatments for illness. Today, the use of Chinese herbal medicines is common among Chinese communities worldwide. Many books on the use of Chinese functional foods for health maintenance purpose have been published in recent years. Information and knowledge in this area, particularly in Chinese publications, are becoming more and more accessible to the general public.

Although Chinese functional foods are generally mild in action and with little or no side effects, caution should be exercised when designing food recipes using Chinese functional ingredients. Like the practice of herbal medicine, basic Chinese medical theories should be used to guide the correct application of these herbal ingredients. Just as in the prescription of Chinese herbal medicine for disease treatment, formulas in the design of functional foods should be tailored to suit individual needs, based on the recipient's body constitution and health condition. Inappropriate use of Chinese functional foods could cause harm. Common examples of misuse of Chinese functional foods include using warm or hot nature herbs for people with a hot type of constitution or disease; or using cool or cold foods for patients with a cold type of condition. Other misuses of functional foods include fortifying the body with large amounts of qi and blood tonics while pathogenic factors such as phlegm and blood stasis are evident in the body. If the use of Chinese functional foods does not conform to Chinese medical principles, it can have detrimental consequences for the patients. It should also be stressed that when using Chinese functional foods, the recipient's basic constitution, underlying disease and other environmental factors, such as season, climate and geographical location, should all be taken into consideration. For example, it is not recommended to incorporate hot type medicinal ingredients such as (*Cervi Cornu Pantotrichum*) *lu rong* and *Zanthoxyli Pericarpium* (*Hua jiao*) as functional foods during the hottest period of summer. By the same token, cold type functional ingredients such as *Taraxaci Herba* (*Pu gong ying*) and *Sophora Flos* (*Huai hua*) should not be incorporated as functional foods in the depths of winter.

From the dawn of history, attempts have been made to retard or mitigate the aging process. Obvious ways of doing so include leading a healthy life style and taking regular exercise, and a balanced diet probably also plays an important role in keeping elderly people fit and young in spirit. Chinese functional foods with anti-aging properties would add an extra dimension for enhancing the general well-being of the aged. Since vacuity of the kidney essence and qi, general decline of bodily visceral functions, and the accumulation of phlegm and blood stagnation are the fundamental reason that drives the aging process, most anti-aging food recipes employ herbs that have kidney tonifying, spleen strengthening and qi supplementing, phlegm dissolving and blood circulation invigorating substances. Several pharmacological properties are thought to be related to the benefits of anti-aging Chinese functional foods, including immuno-stimulating, anti-oxidant, lipid/cholesterol-lowering, neuroprotection and anti-cancer.

It is worth pointing out that the use of the Chinese functional foods for anti-aging or other health promotion purposes is mainly at the ethno-medicinal and ethno-pharmacological levels, and the health benefits and efficacy related to the use of Chinese functional foods are largely anecdotal. Reliable evidence for their claimed health benefits, especially evidence derived from well designed and executed clinical studies, is in short supply. The dearth of reliable evidence is not surprising, as most people use Chinese functional foods privately at home, and the formulas used are invariably diverse, varied and inconsistent. Nevertheless, extensive experience has been accumulated in the use of a wide variety of functional food ingredients for health promotion purpose, and the practice of functional foods in daily living has become a cultural phenomenon. Although concrete evidence regarding their health benefits is patchy, the community-wide observation suggests that certain health benefits are associated with the use of functional foods. Claims that functional foods promote health are to a certain extent strengthened by the fact that the average life expectancies in Hong Kong and Macau, where their citizens widely incorporate Chinese functional foods into their daily cooking, are among the highest in the world. Chinese functional foods will probably become an increasingly popular field of research in the near future. In turn, as more is known about how these foods work, more and more people around the world are likely to adopt the time-honoured Chinese practice of using functional natural ingredients to improve their health.

References

Dang, Y., Peng, Y. and Li, W.K. (1999) *Chinese Functional Food*. New World Press, Beijing.

Deng, H.B., Cui, D.P., Jiang, J.M., Feng, Y.C., Cai, N.S. and Li, D.D. (2003) Inhibiting effects of *Achyranthes bidentata* polysaccaride and *Lycium barbarum* polysaccharide on nonenzyme glycation in D-galactose induced mouse ageing model. *Biomed. Environ. Sci.* **16**, 267–275.

Dai, S., Wen, R. and Li, W. (1994) The values of *Lycium barbarum* to human being in antisenility and prolonging lifespan. *Geriatr. J.* **14**, 33–36.

Jafari, M., Felgner, J.S., Bussel, I.I., Huthili, T., Khodayari, B., Rose, M.R., Vince-Cruz, C. and Mueller, L.D. (2007) Rhodiola: A promising anti-ageing Chinese herb. *Rejuv. Res.* **10**, 587–602.

Jiang, L.D., Zhou, L.Z. and Ma, Y. (2004) Discussion on the relationship of toxicity removing and resolving, life-nurturing and brain health. *Chin. Inform. J. Chin. Med.* 2004, 100–101.

Jiangsu New Medical College (1985) *Encyclopedia of Chinese Materia Medica*. Shanghi Science and Technology Publishing House, Shanghai, P.I.

Lei, H., Wang, B., Li, W.P., Yang, Y., Zhou, A.W. and Chen, M.Z. (2003) Anti-ageing effect of astragalosides and its mechanism of action. *Acta Pharmacologica Sinica* **24**, 230–234.

Li, J. (2005) Understanding ageing from Chinese medicine's perspective. Heilongjiang *Med. J.* **29**, 788–789.

Li, W., Yin, Y., Gong, H., Wu, G. and Zhu, F. (2009) Protective effects of AST and ASI on memory impairment and its mechanism in senescent rats treated by GC. *J. Chin. Herb. Med.* **34**, 199–203.

Li, X.M., Ma, Y.L. and Liu, X.J. (2007) Effect of the Lycium barbarum polysaccharides on age-related oxidative stress in aged mice. *J. Ethnopharmacol.* **111**, 504–511.

Lu, Z.Z. (2001) Chinese medicine presents new opportunity for life nurturing and health preservation for middle-aged and elderly people. *Chin. Healthc Nutr.* **8**, 14.

Luo, Q., Cai, Y., Yan, J., Sun, M. and Corde, H. (2004) Hypoglycemic and hypolipidemic effects and antioxidant activity of fruit extracts from *Lycium barbarum*. *Life Sci.* **76**, 137–149.

McElhaney J.E., Gravenstein, S., Cole S.K., Davidson, E., O'Neill,D., Petitjean, S., Rumble, B. and Shan, J.J. (2004) A placebo-controlled trial of proprietary extract of North American Ginseng (CVT-E002) to prevent acute respiratory illness in institutionalized older adults. *J. Am. Geriatri. Soc.* **52**, 13–19.

Ministry of Health (2002a) List of substances which are both food and medicine. Ministry of Health Ordinance No. 51.

Ministry of Health (2002b) List of substances which can be used as health foods. Ministry of Health Ordinance No. 51.

Nishijo, H., Uwano, T., Zhong, Y.M. and Ono, T. (2004) Proof of the mysterious efficacy of ginseng: Basic and clinical trials: Effects of red ginseng of learning and memory deficits in an animal model of amnesia. *J. Pharmacol. Sci.* **95**, 145–152.

Shen, L.H. and Zhang, J.T. (2004) Ginsenoside Rg1 promotes proliferation of hippocampal progenitor cells. *Neurol. Res.* **26**, 422–428.

Wang, J.H., Wang, H.Z., Zhang, M. and Zhang, S.H. (2002) Anti-ageing function of polysaccharides from *Fructus Lycii*. *Acta Nutr. Sin.* **24**, 189–194.

Wei, X.D., Wang, Z., Shan, H.B., Zhang, P.X. and Ou, Q. (2006) Effects of *astragulus mongholicus* bunge on apoptosis of neurocytes and the expression of relevant gene in the brain of ageing mice. *Chin. J. Clin. Rehabil.* **10**, 151–153.

Yang, T.X. (2002) The relationship of phlegm turbidity in Chinese medicine and ageing. *Hunan J. Tradit Chin. Med.* **8**, 521–522.

Yu, M.S., Leung, S.K.Y., Lai, S.W., Che, C.M., Zee, S.Y., So, K.F., Yuen, W.H. and Chang, R.C.C. (2005) Neuroprotective effects of anti-ageing oriental medicine *Lycium barbarum* against β-amyloid peptide neurotoxicity. *Exp. Gerontol.* **40**, 716–727.

Yu, M.S., Lai, C.S.W., Ho, Y.S., Zee, S.Y., So K.F., Yuen, W.H. and Chang, R.C.C. (2007) Characterization of the effects of anti-ageing medicine *Fructus lycii* on β-amyloid peptide neurotoxicity. *Int. J. Mol. Med.* **17**, 1157–1162.

Yu, Z.Y. (1992). Exploring the mechanisms of ageing in Chinese medicine: The impact of ageing on the pattern of deficiency in the cause and excess in manifestations. *Chin. J. Integr. Chin. West. Med.* **2**, 80.

Zhang, J.G., Yang, N., He, H., Wei, G.H., Gao, D.S., Wang, X.L., Wang, X.Z. and Song, G.Y. (2005) Effect of astragalus injection on plasma levels of apoptosis-related factors in aged patients with chronic heart failure. *Chin. J. Integr. Med.* **11**, 187–190.

Zhao, H., Li, Q., Zhang, Z., Pei, X., Wang, J. and Li, Y. (2009) Long-term ginsenoside consumption prevents memory loss in aged SAMP8 mice by decreasing oxidative stress and up-regulated the plasticity-related proteins in hippocampus. *Brain Res.* **1256**, 111–122.

Chapter 6

Herbal Formulation for Anti-Aging

Song-Ming Liang

Abstract

Huangdi Neijing called the natural life time of human beings "heavenly age"; it was taken as the age that human beings should live and was the highest standard of long life. Modern people, beginning from middle or old age, are influenced not only by the living environment but also by their intrinsic factors and the incidence of many diseases have increased significantly, so that "living to the heavenly age" of human beings is affected. The knowledge about aging in Traditional Chinese Medicine is very rich and it has established a complete series of principles and methods, contributing much to the health care of human beings. This chapter recommends in brief, the drugs and formulae of anti-aging and prolongation of life; and also the procedures of health maintenance and hygiene promotion used in Traditional Chinese Medicine.

Keywords: Anti-Aging; Prolongation of Life; Health Preserving; Hygiene; TCM Drugs.

The life time of human beings is limited. Limitation means the natural age which people can live to. *Huangdi Neijing* called the natural age of human beings as "heavenly age." It meant that human should live to that age and thought that "living to the heavenly age" was the highest standard of long life. For example, from *Neijing Suwen — Real Treatise on the Ancient Heaven*, "The people nowadays have many errors. They drink wine like water, become accustomed to bad habits, have sex in a drunken state, tend to overuse their energy ignorant about the way to keep up their physical and spiritual strength. They chase after unbounded enjoyment, lead a life without harmony and therefore, they are aging at fifty." Of course, besides the above factor affecting the length of life-spans, there are also other reasons, such as, environment, weather, nutrition, mental condition, medical and hygienic condition, economic situation and personal hygiene; all these have influence on health.

There are many ways to delay the occurrence of aging. *Neijing* proposed a complete series of health maintenance and hygiene principles and methods such as health maintenance by regular living habits, by control of the mental status, by appropriate exercises, by medication, etc. This paper emphasizes formulae on TCM drugs and old formulae for health maintenance and retardation of aging under stress.

Disease in old and middle ages is usually due to weakness and lowering of resistance. Weakness in old and middle age people is usually characterized by weakened body resistance, the clinical manifestations of which may be summarized as deficiency of *qi*, deficiency of blood, deficiency of *yin*, deficiency of *yang* — the four types. Due to the inter-dependence of *qi*, blood, *yin* and *yang* on one another, in the condition of deficiency, they also affect one another, so that the syndromes of deficiency of both *qi* and blood, deficiency of both *yin* and *yang*, deficiency of both *qi* and *yang* etc. exist. Therefore, the Chinese medical formulations for health promotion are mostly of the replenishing and strengthening types.

6.1 The Theoretical Basis of Anti-Aging and Health Maintenance Drug in Traditional Chinese Medicine

The recognition of anti-aging is very different between modern medicine and traditional medicine. Scholars in China and abroad, from the modern medicine point of view, have proposed more than ten theories about anti-aging. Those that are commonly accepted are as follows:

(1) Free radical theory (Harman, 1968): with the increase of age, the anti-oxygenation enzyme SOD, GSH-PX decreases in activity and there is accumulation of free radicals which act with the unsaturated fatty acid in the cell membrane to form the hyper-oxygenated lipids (LPO), inducing injures to the cell membrane and further initiation of disease and aging.
(2) Weakening of immune power theory: As age increases, the immune function of the body decreases and there is disorder of the body

equilibrium regulation mechanism, so that the power to fight against disease weakens and the incidence of infection, tumor and immunologic diseases significantly increase.

(3) Lipofuscin accumulation theory: Lipofuscin in the body accumulates gradually as age increases, especially in the cerebral cortex and hippocampus which is an important morphological index in aging of animals. Excess of lipofuscin damages the nerve cell, leads to decrease of cerebral function as well as to the injury of other systems in the body and, finally, to the onset of disease (Qu, 1999).

Aging in TCM was written early in *Huangdi Neijing* and it was thought that the phenomenon of life was based on the function of *Zhang-fu* materials of the body. The body's progression from energetic to weak is chiefly due to the rise and decline of the kidney. Kidney is the root of the *five-zhang* and *six-fu*, is the fundamental of innateness. The essence of kidney can nourish *five-zhang*; kidney generates marrow and the brain is the seat of marrow. The medical literature, through generations, wrote down that TCM drugs for health maintenance and prolongation of age basically belonged to the category of kidney replenishing. From the viewpoint of modern medicine, the kidney replenishing method can regulate the endocrine system, increase the function of sexual gland, regulate immunologic function and enhance the function of the brain (Xu, 1994).

6.2 TCM Drugs and Immunologic Function of the Body

Scientific investigation demonstrates that aging is closely related to the healthy status of the immunologic defense power of human beings and animals. Traditional Chinese Medicine recognizes that the attack of disease is due to "weakened body resistance" and "excess of pathogens". *Huangdi Neijing* states that: The vital-*qi* stays in the interior, pathogens do not invade. and "If pathogen invades, there must be deficiency of *qi*." Vital-*qi* — the defense power of the body and regulatory function; it summarizes the normal function of the immunologic system of the body. Clinical and laboratory studies demonstrate that in most patients, their immune functions are lower than normal or show disturbance, and the application of drugs to replenish deficiency can cause increase or normalization of immune function. Also, some drugs for clearing away heat and toxic material or for promoting blood circulation to remove blood stasis can induce regulation of immune function in different diseases. In the differentiation of deficiency syndrome, most of the cases belong to the deficiency of lung, spleen and kidney, showing a decrease of immune function, especially in cases of the deficiency of kidney. Most of the replenishing drugs for deficiency and a small amount of the drugs removing pathogens are effective in promoting the immune function.

The replenishing and strengthening drugs include the effect of invigorating *qi*, enriching the blood, invigorating *yin* and invigorating *yang*.

Invigorating *qi*
Drugs — ginseng, astragalus root, pilose asiabelt root, lucid ganoderma, atrocitylodes liquorices, mushroom species.
Formulae — *Sijunzi* decoction, *Buzhong yiqi* decoction, *Shengmai san*, *Yupingfeng* powder.

Enriching blood
Drugs — *Angelica sinensis*, prepared rehmannia root, white peony root, donkey-hide gelatin, *Millettia reticulata* Benth.
Formulae — *Siwu* decoction *Danggui Buxue Tang*.

Invigorating *yin*
Drugs — wolfberry fruit, ophiopogon root, locid asparagus, dendrobium, *huanggui*, tremella, adenophora root, *Ligustrum lucidum*.
Formulae — *Liuwei Dihuang Wan*, *Erzhi* pills, *Zuogui* decoction.

Invigorating *yang*
Drugs — Dodder seed, epimedium, morinda root, desert living cistanche, pilose antler, psoralea fruit, *Cordyceps sinensis*.
Formulae — *Shenqi Wan*, *Yougui* decoction (*wan*).

Drugs for eliminating pathogens include the drugs to clear heat, drugs to invigorate spleen for eliminating dampness by diuresis and also drugs for promotion of blood circulation and removal of blood stasis.

Drugs for clearing heat — *Radix scutellariae*, *Rhizoma coptidis* cortex phellodendri, *Herba hedyotis*, common Andrographis herb.
Drugs to invigorate spleen for eliminating dampness — umbellate pore, poria, coix seed

Drugs for promotion of blood circulation and removal of blood stasis — Sichuan lovage rhizome, safflower.

These drugs are related to the promotion of immunity and regulation of body function. They exert their influences only when the body is in a state of "excess syndrome" with lowering of the immune function. Therefore, without syndrome differentiation, one should not use them as a routine to promote immune function in cases requiring elimination of pathogens; especially in using the drugs bitter in taste and cold in nature, drugs for resolution of blood stasis or toxic drugs, one must be careful.

In the 360 herbal drugs stated in *Shennong Bencao Jing*, 165 species were known that they could "lighten the body and prolong the age" and among them many only had a cosmetic effect. With the progress of modern medical pharmacology research, however, it has been proven that many natural TCM herbal drugs really do have the pharmacological action of delaying the process of growing old.

The herbal drugs for delaying aging in the *Shennong Bencao Jing* are as follows:

The superior ones:

Ginseng: long term taking can lighten the body and prolong life.

Lucid asparagus: long term taking can lighten the body and prolong life.

Liquorice: long term taking can lighten the body and prolong life.

Dried rehmannia root: long term taking can lighten the body and prolong life.

Atractylodes rhizome: long term taking can lighten the body, prolong life and resist hunger.

Dodder seed: long term taking can brighten the eyes, lighten the body and prolong life.

Bidentata: long term taking can lighten the body and endure aging.

Rhizoma Polygonati Odorati: long term taking can remove blackness and dryness of face, refine facial complexion, lighten the body and prolong life.

Ophiopogon root: long term taking can lighten the body, delay oldness and resist hunger.

Chinese yam: long term taking enable better sight and hearing, can lighten the body, resist hunger and prolong life.

Coix seed: long term taking can lighten the body and replenish *qi*.

Polygola root: long term taking can lightem the body and delay aging.

Dendrobium: long term taking can strengthen the stomach and intestines, lighten the body and prolong life.

Gordon everyale seed: long term taking can resist hunger, delay aging and lighten the body.

Ganoderma lucidum: long term taking can lighten the body, delay aging and prolong life.

Desertliving cistanche: long term taking can lighten the body.

Wolfberry fruit: long term taking can strengthen the bones and tendons, lighten the body and delay aging.

Poria: long term taking can stabilize the soul, tranqulize the mind, resist hunger and prolong life.

Eucommia bark: long term taking can lighten the body and be able to endure aging.

Ligustrum: long term taking can strengthen and lighten the body and delay aging.

Donkey-hide gelatin: long term taking can lighten the body and replenish *qi*.

Tortoise plastron: long term taking can lighten the body and resist hunger.

Chinese-date: long term taking can lighten the body.

Sesami Nigrum Semen: long term taking can delay aging.

The drugs of the middle grade include the following:

Dogwood fruit: long term taking can lighten the body.

Umbellate pore: long tem taking can lighten the body and be able to endure aging.

Longan aril: long term taking can strengthen the soul, have better sight and hearing, lighten the body, delay aging and he able to communicate with God.

Silktree albizia bark: can make one feeling happy and carefree, long term taking can lighten the body, brighten sight and get things as one wishes.

Some classic TCM formulae have also the effect of delaying aging.

Shengmai san, introduced by the famous physician Li Dong Yuan in the *Yuan Dynasty* in the book *Treatise on Differentiation of Problems in Internal and External Damage.*

Ingredients: ginseng, ophiopogon root, schisandra fruit.

Indication:

> *Original* indication: in the late stage of summer-heat showing the syndrome of injury of *qi* and *yin.*
>
> *Present indication*: in miscellaneous diseases showing syndrome of injury of *qi* and *yin* of the lung and spleen or when the patient has chronic cough with the syndrome of injury of *qi* and *yin.*

Formula:

> *Sovereign drug* — ginseng: replenishing *qi* of the heart, spleen and lung.
>
> *Minister drug* — Ophiopogon root: nourishing *yin* (the *yin* of heart, lung and stomach), promoting production of the body fluid (stomach fluid).
>
> *Assistant and envoy drug* — schisandra fruit: promoting the production of body fluid (stomach fluid), assisting the lung (*qi*), relieving cough and suppressing sweating.

Modern investigation has revealed that *Shengmai san* can increase immunologic power of the body, improve myocardial function, enhance absorption and digestion, raise the activity of the whole body, nourish and strengthen the body, prevent fatigue and promote anti-aging. It can also be applied to treat shock, especially the kinds of shock resulting from injury of *qi* and *yin.* This formula has a strong effect on the elevation of blood pressure. There are preparations for intravenous injection for emergency use in shock. It was stated in *Collection and Explanations on Medical Formulae*: "when a patient was dying and the pulse not palpable, if given this formula, he could be alive. Its therapeutic effect was really great and therefore, it was called *Shengmai san* (the pulse alive powder)." It is usually used in obstinate insomnia of the *qi* and *yin* deficiency type with some effectiveness.

The *Tortoise and Deer gelatin* (soft extract), introduced in the *Ming Dynasty* (in the year 1569) in the book *Briefs in Medicine* by Wang Shan Chai.

Ingredients: deer-horn gelatin, tortoise plastron, ginseng, wolfberry fruit.

Therapeutic effect: nourishing *yin* and strengthening *yang*, replenishing *qi* and enriching blood.

Indication: deficiency type of injury of vitality syndrome of deficiency of *yin* and blood (deficiency of *qi*, blood, *yin* and *yang*).

Formula:

> *Sovereign drug* — Deer-horn gelatin: warmly strengthen the kidney *yang* (replenishing *yang*). It is a passionate product with blood and flesh; it replenishes the essence of life and restores the marrow.
>
> *Tortoise-plastron gelatin*: a passionate product with blood and flesh, replenishes the essence of life and restores the marrow, nourishes *yin* and enriches blood.
>
> *Minister and assistant drug* — ginseng: replenishing and supplementing the *qi* middle-*jiao* (replenishing *qi*); Wolfberry fruit: replenishing and supplementing *yin* and blood (supplementing blood).

This formula nourishes and replenishes *qi* and blood as well as *yin* and *yang*, and is used in patients showing deficiency of *qi* and blood. In modern times it is used to treat underdevelopment caused by endocrine disorder severe anemia, neurosis and decrease of sexual function which belong to the category of deficiency of *yin*, *yang*, *qi* and blood.

Qibao meiran mini-pills, introduced in the book *"Collected Exegesis of Recipes."*

Ingredients: fleece-flower root, poria, bidentata, Chinese angelica root, wolfberry fruit, dodder seed, psoralea fruit.

Therapeutic effect: replenishing and supplementing the liver and kidney, enriching blood and blackening the hair.

Indication: deficiency of liver and kidney and deficiency of essence and blood causing premature whitening of hair, loosening of teeth, soreness of loin, seminal emission and premature ejaculation and deficiency of kidney causing infertility.

Formula:

> *Sovereign drug* — Fleece flower root: as the most important drug to supplement liver and kidney and replenish essence and blood.

Minister drug — Chinese angelica root, wolfberry fruit: helps the monarch drug to replenish essence and blood and blacken the hair.

Assistant and envoy drug — Dodder seed, psoralea fruit, and bidentate: help the monarch drug to supplement liver and kidney; Poria: strengthen the spleen, promote diuresis and gives the formula a replenishing character but has no stagnating effect.

This formula supplements the liver and kidney with a median force and is effective in whitening of hair in the middle age, in baldness, oligospermia and male infertility Laboratory research demonstrated that this formula, under anoxic condition, can raise the responsive and survival ability of the body. Clinical studies showed that *Qibao meiran mini-pills* can lessen the damage to the body caused by the free radical, raise the disturbance of lipid metabolism and endocrine hormone level. These actions cause the supplement of kidney and strengthening of *yang* and promote anti-aging and health preserving and also prolongation of life (Cao, 2006).

Shouwu Yanshou pills, introduced in the book *Shibuzhai Medical Book*.
Ingredients: fleece-flower root, polyporous grass, mulberry, black sesame, Cherokee rose-hip, eclipta, dodder seed, ligustrum, bidentata mulberry leaf, honey suckle flower, eucommia bark.
Therapeutic effect — supplementing liver and kidney, enriching essence and blood, strengthening the bone and tendons and whitening of hair.
Indication — Insufficiency of liver and kidney, deficiency of body essence and blood causing dizziness and dim eyesight, tinnitus, hard of hearing, numbness of limbs, weakness of loin and knees, nocturnal diuresis, premature whitening of hair and beard.
Formula:
Sovereign drug — Fleece-flower root: emphatically prescribed to supplement liver and kidney and to replenish the body essence and blood.
Minister drug — ligustrum, eclipta, mulberry, black sesame, eucoamia bark, polyporous grass, bidentata all help the monarch drug to nourish and supplement the liver and kidney and enrich the body essence and blood.
Assistant and envoy drugs — Cherokee rose-hip: reinforcing the kidney and controlling nocturnal emission, mulberry leaf, honeysuckle flower: clearing away heat.

This formula is applied to patients suffering from deficiency of *yin* of the liver and kidney, insufficient body essence and blood together with symptoms of heat showing bitterness of mouth and dryness of throat or showing tidal fever. It can lower the level of cholesterol, decrease the formation of plaques on the intima of arteries and the deposition of fat (Wang *et al.*, 2002).

6.3 Important Classical Health Preserving Anti-Aging Formulae

In Traditional Chinese Medicine, the research literature about anti-aging is very abundant. There are many formula studied which belong to, according to their effectiveness, chiefly the following three categories: replenishing kidney, strengthening spleen, activating blood and removal of stasis

(1) Formula for replenishing *qi* and anti-aging *Sijunzi decoction* (for-mula from *Taiping Huimin Heji Ju Fang*).

Ingredients: pilose asiabell root atractylodes rhizome, poria, pre-pared licorice.

Therapeutic effect: replenishing *qi* and strengthening spleen.

Indication: syndrome of deficiency of spleen, stomach and *qi*.

Formula:

Sovereign drug — pilose asiabell root: supplementing *qi* and strengthening spleen.

Minister drug — atractylodes rhizome: helps the monarch drug in supplementing *qi* and strengthening spleen and can also promote dryness with bitter taste to overcome dampness of the spleen because the spleen is fond of dryness and hates dampness.

Assistant drug — poria: strengthening spleen and promoting diure-sis, making this formula good for supplement but causing no stagna-tion, prepared liquorices assist pilose asiabell root and atractylodes rhizome in supplementing *qi* and strengthening spleen.

Envoy drug — prepared liquorice: regulating the properties of drugs.

The four drugs in this formula have the property of acting independently, they are not hot and not dry, they supplement calmly, not using excessive force, and act justly without deviation and because of their noble behavior, the formula is called *Decoction of four Noble Drugs*. It is a basic formula for treating deficiency of *qi* of the spleen and stomache. If taken in adequate amounts, it is not only helpful in the regulation of the nervous system, improvement of the cell metabolism of the gastric mucous membrane, and restoration of the disturbed gastrointestinal function, but also comparatively effective in chronic indigestion, chronic enteritis and peptic ulcer. It is also effective in supplementing *qi*, strengthening the body, in anti-aging and prolongation of life; it is beneficial in the above conditions when taken in long term (Zhong *et al.*, 2009).

Huang qi tang introduced from *Sheng Ji Zong Lu.*
Ingredients: astragalus root, pilose asiabell root, atractylodes rhizome, bark of Chinese cassia tree, fresh ginger, Chinese: date.
Therapeutic effect: invigorating *qi* and strengthening the spleen; warming *yang* and eliminating coldness.
Indication: deficiency and coldness syndrome of spleen and stomach.
Formula:

> *Sovereign drug* — astragalus root: invigorating *qi* and strengthening the spleen.
>
> *Minister drug* — pilose assiabell root: helps the Sovereign drug to invigorate *qi* and strengthen the spleen; atratylodes rhizome: helps the monarch drug to invigorate *qi* and strengthen the spleen and through dryness and bitter tasting to overcome dampness of the spleen.
>
> *Assistant drug* — Chinese-date: assisting the monarch and ministerial drugs to invigorate *qi* and strengthen the spleen; bark of Chinese cassia fresh tree and fresh ginger: warming *yang* and invigorating pulse-beat, cooperating with invigorating drugs to give the result of warming without dryness and promoting smooth circulation of *qi* and blood.
>
> *Envoy drug* — Chinese date: regulate the action of drugs.

The astragalus root decoction can significantly increase the immunologic power of the body, regulate gastrointestinal and endocrine function, enhance digestive absorption, strengthen the body muscles and prevent deposition of lipid and metabolic products. If taken in appropriate amounts, it has the effect of anti-aging.

(2)   Formulae for enriching blood and anti-aging *Siwu decoction* from
      the book "*Secret Formulae Endowed by Fairy about Healing Trauma
      and Continuation of the Broken*."
      Ingredients: prepared rehmannia root, Chinese angelica root, white
      peony root chuanxiong rhizome.
      Therapeutic effect: enriching and activating blood.
      Indication: deficiency of blood and stasis of blood syndrome.
      Formula:
      Sovereign drug — prepared rehmannia root: nourishing *yin* and
      enriching blood.
      Minister drug — Chinese angelica root: enriching and activating
      blood, regulate menstruation and relieving dysmenorrhea.
      Assistant and envoy drug — white peony root: helps the monarch
      and ministerial drug to replenish blood and nourish *yin*.
      Chuanxiong rhizome: helps Chinese angelica root in activating blood
      and in promoting the circulation of *qi*.

This formula was originally used to treat pain in blood stasis in trauma. Up
to *Taiping Huimin Heji Ju Fang*, its usage was further expanded to many
gynecologic conditions and become a basic formula in replenishing blood
and regulating menstruation. It improves the moving of blood in a circular
way in the body, increases the resistance to anoxia, inhibits the formation
of embolus and therefore results in the therapeutic effect of enriching and
activating blood (Wen *et al.*, 1997).

Danggui Buxue Tang from *Treatise on Differentiation of Problems in
Internal and External Damage*.
Ingredients: astragalus root, Chinese angelica root.
Therapeutic effect: replenishing *qi* and promoting regeneration of
      blood.
Indication: syndrome of deficiency of blood and appearance of fever;
      syndrome of deficiency of *qi* and blood.
Formula:
      Sovereign drug — astragalus root: used to replenish greatly the *qi* of
      spleen and in order to form a source for the regeneration of *qi* and
      blood and for the aim of "regeneration of *yang* goes with rising up of
      yin; prosperity of *qi* leads to regeneration of blood."

Minister and Assistant drug — Chinese angelica root: replenishing blood and giving harmony to nourishment.

Danggui Buxue Tang can raise the immunologic power of the body, improve blood circulation and regulate hormone secretion. Taken in appropriate amount, it has the therapeutic effect of anti-aging (Liu *et al.*, 2005).

6.4 Formula for Supplementing *Yin* and Delay of Aging

Liuwei Dihuang Wan, introduced in the *Song Dynasty* by Qian Yi in the book *Direct Comments on Pediatric Syndrome and Drugs*.
Ingredients: prepared rehmannia root, dogwood fruit, moutan bark, poria, alisma orientalis, Chinese yam.
Therapeutic effect: nourishing and replenishing the kidney *yin*.
Indication: syndrome of deficiency of kidney *yin*.
Formula:

> *Sovereign drug* — prepared rehmannia root: nourish and supplement kidney *yin* filling the body essence and replenishing the marrow.
> *Minister drug* — dogwood fruit; nourishing the liver *yin*.
> Chinese yam: replenishing the spleen *yin*; coordination of the above three drugs produces nourishment of liver, spleen and kidney, customarily called "the three supplements," of which, supplement of kidney is the main part.
> *Assistant and envoy drugs* — poria: assisting Chinese yam to strengthen the spleen; *alisma orientalis*: preventing the grease of prepared rehmannia root. These two drugs both have diuretic effect and can be used to treat unsmooth urination caused by deficiency of kidney.
> *Cortex* moutan: can hinder the dampness and astringent character of dogwood fruit, purge away the kidney fire so that it is effective in treatment of the fire of deficiency type resulting frame deficiency of *yin*.
> Coordination of these three drugs has the effect of purging away dampness, facilitating clearance of the fire of deficiency type which is customarily called "the three purgatives."

Liuwei dihuang wan, in the present time, is commonly used to treat chronic nephritis, hypertension, diabetes pulmonary tuberculosis, hyperthyroidism, climacteric syndrome, etc. It has also a good regulatory effect on disorders of the autonomic nervous system (Wu, 2009).

Er Zhi Wan from *Collected Exegesis of Recipes*
Ingredients: ligustrum, eclipta.
Therapeutic effect: nourishing the liver and kidney.
Indication: syndrome of deficiency of *yin* of the liver and kidney.
Formula:

>*Sovereign drug* — ligustrum: nourishing the *yin* of the liver and kidney placing stress on supplement of kidney *yin*.
>*Minister and assistant drugs* — eclipta: assisting the monarch drug to nourish the liver and kidney *yin* with a tendency to stress on nourishing liver *yin*.

In this formula, it is better for ligustrum collected on the *Winter Solstice Day* and for eclipta on the *Summer Solstice Day* and so it is called *Er Zhe Wan*. These two drugs both have a better effect on nourishing the liver and kidney, whitening the hair and brightening the eyesight and also they give effective results in dim sight of eyes, tinnitus and premature whitening of hair. If taken in appropriate amounts, it can balance *yin* and *yang* of the kidney, delay aging and prolong life (Xi *et al.*, 2009).

6.5 Formulas for Supplementing *Yang* and Anti-Aging

Shenqi Wan from *"Synopsis of Golden Chamber"*.
Ingredients: dried rehmannia root, dogwood fruit, Chinese yam, alisma orientalis poria, moutan bark prepared aconite root, cinnamom twig.
Therapeutic effect: replenishing warmly the kidney *yang*.
Indication: syndrome of deficiency of kidney *yang*.
Formula:

>*Sovereign drug* — prepared aconite root cinnamom twig; promoting circulation of qi and expulsion of water, slight activation of blood circulation; the two drugs both have the effect of warming the kidney and promoting *yang*.
>*Minister drug* — dried rehmannia root: nourishing the kidney *yin* dogwood fruit: nourishing the liver *yin*. Chinese yam: tonifying and nourishing the spleen *yin*.

Assistant and envoy drugs — poria: also assisting Chinese yam to strengthen the spleen.

Alisma orientalis: also preventing the grease of prepared rehmannia root.

Cortex moutan: also preventing the dampness and astringent character of dogwood fruit.

Shenqi Wan is really a prescription which can invigorate both *yin* and *yang*, and therefore can be used in the syndrome of deficiency of both *yin* and *yany*; it can improve the function of pituitary adrenocortex as well as the function of kidney. If taken in appropriate amounts, it is not only effective in middle and old age chronic nephritis, diabetes, disorders of the autonomic nervous system, dementia and early stage prostatic hypertrophy, but also effective in replenishing the spleen, nourishing the liver, strengthening the body and prolongation of life (Zhang, 2009).

Mijing wan, introduced from *Standards for Diagnosis and Treatment*
Ingredients: prepared aconite root, desertliving cistanche, morinda root, bidentata, calcining dragon's bone.
Therapeutic effect: warming the kidney and strengthening *yang*, promoting astringency of semen.
Indication: syndrome of deficiency and coldness of kidney *yang* and inability of controlling the ejaculation of semen.
Formula:

Sovereign drug — prepared aconite root: warming the kidney and strengthening *yang*

Minister drug — morinda root, desertliving cistanche: assisting the monarch drug to warm and strengthen kidney *yang*; Calcining dragon's bone: promote astringency of semen

Assistant and envoy drug — bidentata: assisting morinda root and desertliving cistanche to supplement the liver and kidney and strengthen the bone and tendons.

Mijing wan is effective in promoting blood circulation and improvement of kidney function. Taken in appropriate amounts, it is effective in seminal emission, impotence, intolerance of cold, coldness of limbs and freezing pain of the loin and knees in middle and old age people suffering from deficiency of kidney *yang*. It can warm and replenish the fire from the gate of life and regulate the kidney *yin* and *yang* to stay in a balanced condition so as to attain the aim of anti-aging and prolongation of life.

6.6 Health Maintenance in Traditional Chinese Medicine

Health maintenance is a learning which studies strengthening of the body to prevent disease and to prolong life. The Chinese nation had a long history and culture of health maintenance which promoted the prosperous development of the nation.

Health is the most precious property in the life process of human beings as, without health, nothing can be done, and things such as learning, employment success would all lose their meaning. The World Health Organization (WHO) proposed that there are four factors critical to health: (1) intrinsic factor heredity 15%, (2) extrinsic factors 17% (social environment 10%, natural environment 6%; and (3) medical condition 8% (4) personal lifestyle 60%. From the above we know that the health of human beings is critically related to the lifestyle of the individual. Health maintenance teaches us the correct lifestyle; it is an important way to achieve good health. Later, WHO added regular living habit as one of the basic elements in health maintenance: i.e. reasonable diets 25%, adequate exercises and restriction from smoking and wine drinking 25% psychological balance 50%. According to the social welfare Department of America, using the medical method, in spite of spending millions or even billions of money, the number of predate deaths decreased only 10%, while using the preventive health maintenance methods, without spending much money, the predate deaths decreased 70%. This demonstrated the extreme importance of health maintenance.

From the TCM point of view, through various ways of protecting health, that is health maintenance, we can increase the body constitution to a higher level and enhance the power of resisting disease and the response ability of vital *qi* to the external, environment, and, hence, decrease the chance of being attacked by diseases. This is to say that the life process of an individual is in a state of regulation of *yin* and *yang*, there is harmony of the body, his (her) health and psychological status is in the best condition, so that the chance of being attacked by cancer is decreased and the aging process is delayed. Therefore, for the prevention of disease, increase of human health standards and for prolongation of life, health preserving is extremely important.

1. Time sequence of health maintenance

Time sequence of health preserving is also called health maintenance by sequence of four seasons. It means that human beings should adapt themselves to the changes of seasons and to the regulation of the interchange of *yin* and *yang*, so that they can regulate their diets and living habits and let the body to suit the natural environment and this is the so-called "heaven and mankind blended into one".

Neijing, under the theory of "heaven and man kind blended into one" and "four season's *five-zhang* and *yin yang*," acknowledged that "The four seasons and *yin yang* are the fundamentals of all materials, so that wise men nourish *yang* in spring and summer, and nourish *yin* in autumn and winter." It therefore proposed the concept of health maintenance in time sequence and according to the theory of regulation of the mind in the four seasons, arranged the health maintenance methods in spring, summer, autumn and winter.

6.6.1 *Health maintenance in spring*

In daily life one should be aware of taking on enough clothes, keeping warm and avoid getting cold. There is a poem, saying: "Do not take off your cotton padded clothes in February, there is still snow like pear flower in March." Spring is coming from winter and especially in early spring, the temperature is sometimes cold and sometimes warm. Besides, spring dominates wind and wind is abundant during spring.

The diet should be beneficial to the spleen and include the drugs such as Chinese yam, gordon euryale seed, and lotus seed. Spring belongs to liver wood and when liver *qi* is abundant, it may be overloaded and then one should take drugs which can protect the liver, like chrysanthemum flower, prunella spike abrus cantoniensis, wolfberry fruit, etc. One should restrain from taking oily, fried, roasted, peppery or very hot food, or food hard to be digested to avoid accumulation of fire internally and activation of liver fire. Sour food may evoke excessive production of liver *qi* (sourness goes into the liver) and therefore one should take less sour food.

Soup for strengthening spleen and eliminating indigestion is the health preserving soup in spring. Its ingredients are: hawthorn fruit, parch germinated barley, each five *qian*, tangerine peel two *qian*, decoct with water.

Therapeutic effect: strengthening the spleen and whetting the appetite, soothing the liver and regulating the flow of *qi*. It is indicated in indigestion, fullness of stomach and distension of abdomen.

6.6.2 *Health maintenance in summer*

In summer, the weather is hot and damp, clothes should be good for absorbing sweat, easy for passing in of air and be thin, light, spacious and comfortable. One should take a nap for half an hour to eliminate fatigue and restore physical strength.

In the hot summer weather, dampness may be severe; the body sweats easily, consumes body fluid and hurts *yin*. The diet should be heat-clearing and the food easy to eat. There are food having the character of sweet and cool facilitating the increase of body fluid, relieving summer heat and promoting diuresis, such as watermelon and mung bean. One should restrain from taking oily, fried and indigestible food. Those with too cold character should not be taken too frequently. One of the summer health maintenance soups is the wax gourd, coix seed, mung bean soup. Its ingredients are: wax gourd (half *jin*), coix seed and mung bean each two *liang*. Boil the soup and eat the beans. Therapeutic effect, clearing away summer-heat and promoting diuresis, indicated in hot summer weather to relieve vexation and thirst.

6.6.3 *Health maintenance in autumn*

In autumn, it is not suitable to add clothes too early because early autumn has just come from summer and the hot weather has not completely disappeared and the adding of clothes should the adequate. The weather welcomes cool gradually after "white Dew" and this is the so-called "the night of 'white Dew' and 'autumnal equinox', becoming cooler night after night." In autumn daily life, clothes should be added or taken off according to characteristics of early autumn and late autumn. The weather is dry in autumn and inside the room, an adequate degree of temperature and humidity should be kept.

The diet should include more moistening food. In early autumn, one should take more moistening food such as horse hoof fruit, pear, sugar cane, etc. In late autumn, one should take moistening food like peanut, walnut orange, sweet potato and wolfberry fruit. One should restrain from pepping hot food like ginger, onion, garlic and fried food.

The lily bulb lung moistening soup is introduced as one of the health preserving soup in autumn. Its ingredients include: lily bulb, adenophora root each one *liang*, pig lung half *jin*; stewed together and flavoured. Drink the soup, eat the meat and the cooked medicinal herbs. Therapeutic effect; nourishing yin and moistening lung indicated in cough from lung dryness, restlessness and discomfort over the heart and chest and dryness of the throat.

6.6.4 *Health maintenance in winter*

"During winter, coldness hurts and when spring comes, diseases are due to warmth." The weather in winter is cold and one should put on more clothes to keep warm and to prevent the attack of common cold. The diet should include more invigorating food to warm the kidney *yang*, for example, beef mutton, chicken and stew foods. Invigorating the kidney essence, strengthening the body constitution and elevating the resistance to disease can achieve the aim of having little or no chance of being attacked by febrile diseases in the coming spring. One should restrain from taking peppery hot food so as to avoid damage to the kidney-essence.

Among the health maintenance soup, there is the *Hetao Bushen Tang*. Its ingredients are: peachseed one *liang*, morinda root and eucommia bark each five *qian*, pilose asiabell root one *liang*. This has the therapeutic effect of replenishing the kidney and reinforcing the loin, supplementing *qi* and strengthening the spleen. It is indicated in deficiency syndrome of both spleen and kidney, soreness and weakness of loin and knees, fatigue and frequent nocturnal urination.

2. Regulation of the mental state and health maintenance
Neijing stated: "One dies if mentality is lost, and survives if gained". It emphasized on the importance of regulation of the mental state in health

preserving. Mentality, here, demotes the spiritual consciousness and thinking activity of an individual. Its concrete parts include:

(1) Keeping quietness and enclosing the spirit.
     Neijing stated: "Quietness facilities residence of the spirit and rest-
     lessness enhances its vanishing." Quietness here means that people
     must keep a tranquil spiritual status, a happy, modest and unselfish
     realm of thought, and, at the same time should restrain from rep-
     utation and materialistic temptation. In this way, one would attain
     the goal of quietness and enclosure of spirit, whereby the vital *qi*
     is not hurt, the resistance to disease is powerful and the strength of
     anti-aging is good." *Neijing* stated: "Tranquility and no request, the
     vital *qi* is with you the spirit resides internally then, how can disease
     invade?" This is a famous idiom of health maintenance.
(2) Change of passion and alteration of character.
     Change of passion means that one's thinking focuses on another
     place or one's love and worry has changed and transferred to other
     things. Alteration of character indicates the correction of wrong
     ideas, adverse feelings or living habits or a controlled expulsion of
     unhealthy passion for the recovery of a happy and calm mood.
         Modern medicine acknowledges that disease, especially cancer,
     is closely related to the decrease of immune ability, and the mental
     state and psychological condition influence the immune ability at all
     times. If an individual, in daily life, is under great mental suppres-
     sion, or psychologically in a depressed condition for a long time,
     the tendency to be attacked by disease (including cancer) is obvious.
     This coincides with the saying of *Neijing*: "One's *qi* must be deficient
     if overcome by evil". One should keep a calm mental state, refrain
     from the desire of personal fame and, gain and when facing unhappy
     events, can maintain a mental equilibrium and, optimistic attitude.
     Thus, one can achieve the goal of having less attacks of illness.
(3) Health maintenance by physical exercise.
     Life depends on moving of the body. Doing regular physical exercise
     can strengthen the body constitution, increase resistance to disease,
     promote health and prolong life. The famous educationist Yan Xi
     Zhai of *Qing Dynasty* stated; "Nothing is better than moving of the

body in keeping fit." There are many ways in physical exercises, like rope skipping, walking, running and gymnastics. For middle and old age people, the traditional Chinese gymnastics is the most appropriate. It includes *taijiquan, baduanjin* and various kinds of *qi gong* and *wushu*, especially *taijiguan* which is the most popular. This kind of Chinese boxing is characterized by its soft and relaxing movements, especially suitable for physically weak individuals. Walking is also an appropriate physical exercise for middle and old age people.

(4) Dietary health maintenance.

The contents of dietary health maintenance are numerous; its main principles are as follows:

   (a) pay attention to dietetic hygiene, prevent unclean food and drinks, avoid eating putrid food;

   (b) advocate a regular diet, cultivate good eating habits, eat at a fixed time and with a fixed quantity, avoid eating too much in a meal or eating in alternation of fullness and hunger; and

   (c) overcome partiality for a particular kind of food.

(5) In taking a medical diet of health maintenance, one must also pay attention to the drug characteristics and channel tropism.

The above mentioned methods of health maintenance had already been written in "*Huangdi Neijing*," It stated "People in ancient times ran a regulated life with a regulated diet; they did not work disorderly and therefore their bodies were in harmony with the mind. They lived to the heavenly age and died one hundred years old." People of today realize that the best mental state is tranquility, the best physical exercise is walking, the best clinician is oneself, the best drug is time (prevention and spontaneous cure) and the best constitution is healthiness.

The discussion on aging is abundant in traditional Chinese Medicine and such literature in ancient China was most plentiful. At present, researches of anti-aging in TCM find out that the chief cause of aging is deficiency of "spleen" and "kidney." Analyzing the TCM formulas used for anti-aging during the recent ten years, it has been found that has the main ones are those of the "kidney replenishing" and/or "spleen replenishing types", comprising 86% of the total (Qu *et al.*, 1995).

Entering the 21st century, human beings enjoy the great progress of social prosperity and while benefited by the scientific and technological development they are also embarrassed by various problems brought about in parallel by the rapid developments. The health of mankind is facing a new challenge. Aging of the population is becoming a serious social and health management problem. Health and longevity is the general desire of mankind. TCM, owning a long history, embraces rich principles and practices of health maintenance. The rich collections of wisdom, from the health maintenance principles of *"Huangdi Neijing"* to the modern TCM anti-aging researches, new fundings have greatly enriched modern geriatrics. Facing the present challenge of anti-aging in all communities, they are expected to make great contribution.

References

Cao Shuang-Yan. (2006) Clinical study of *Qibaomeirandan* on anti-aging effectiveness. *Chin. J. Trauma Disabil. Med.* **14**(3), 41–43.

Harman, D. (1968) Free radical theory of aging: effect of free radical reaction inhibitors on the mortality rate of male LAF mice. *J. Gerontol.* **23**(4), 476–482.

Liu B.-C., Liu L., Wang Y.-L., Chen G.-G., and Wei P. (2005) Recent status of *danggui buxue tang* pharmacological research. *J. Gansu Coll. Tradit. Chin. Med.* **22**(5), 48–50.

Qu L.-S. (1999) Current research status and prospect of anti-aging study with integrated tradition Chinese medicine and western medicine (part one). *J. Guiyang Coll. Tradit. Chin. Med.* **21**(1), 50–51.

Qu Yan-hui, Zhang Liu-tong, and Mei Jia–Jun. (1995) The formation and development of aging mechanism in traditional Chinese medicine. *Guangming J. Chin. Med.* **6**, 1–3.

Wang Gui-Ming and Wu Xiu-Qing. (2002) Experimental study of *shouwu yanshou dan* in anti-aging research on vascular endothelial cell. *Chin. Arch. Tradit. Chin. Med.* **20**(3), 314–315.

Wen Zhi-Bin, Li Jun-Cheng, He Xiao-Fan, *et al.* (1997) Effects of *Siwu Tang* on experimental thrombosis. *Chin. Crit. Care Med.* **9**(3), 139–142.

Wu Xiang-Wen. (2009) Mechanism study and clinical application of *liu wei di huang wan*. *J. Liaoning Univ. Tradit. Chin. Med.* **11**(2), 19–20.

Xi Jun and Tong L. (2009) Recent Status in pharmacological studies of *er zhi wan*. *China Foreign Med. Treat.* **21**, 98–99.

Xu Y.-X. (1994) Experiences of anti-aging drug research. *West China J. Pharmaceut. Sci.* **9**(2), 130.

Zhang Zhao. (2009) Research progress of clinical trial and experimental study on *jinkuishenqiwan* and *youguiwan*. *Liaoning J. Tradit. Chin. Med.* **36**(6), 1049–1051.

Zhong Chun, Zhang Chun-Gang and Zhang Zi-Wen. (2009) Effects of *si junzi* decoction on CD4+T cells in the gastric mucosa of the aging rat. *J. Yichun Coll.* **31**(4), 54–56.

Chapter 7

Chinese Herbal Medicine: Perspectives on Age-Related Neurodegenerative Diseases

Khaled Radad, Rudolf Moldzio, Lin-Lin Liu and Wolf-Dieter Rausch

Abstract

People in different societies have known tremendous of indigenous medicinal plants since prehistoric time. Among these societies, Chinese people have discovered thousands plants of medicinal properties since thousands of years. They have used them in their food and prescriptions to invigorate their body functions and to treat different ailments, respectively. Since the middle of last century, great attention has been paid globally to medicinal plants trying to use their active ingredients as an alternative medicine. During this period, many molecular ingredients have been identified and isolated from these plants by the aid of modern analytical tools. More recently, some of these molecular substances have been shown to exert neuroprotective effects against a number of neurodegenerative disorders by modulating certain CNS targets. This chapter will address and discuss the effect of the most popular Chinese herbs and their active ingredients against age-related neurodegenerative diseases with special references to Alzheimer's and Parkinson diseases.

Keywords: Aging; Alzheimer's Disease; Chinese Herbs; *Ginkgo Biloba*; Neurodegeneration; Neuroprotection; *Panax Ginseng*; Parkinson Disease.

7.1 Introduction

Aging is a term for a set of processes that contribute to age-related decline in performance, productivity and health. Aged populations are continuously rising and approximately 30% of the population will be aged 65 years or older within the next 50 years (Youdim and Joseph, 2001). Aging can be "universal" or "probabilistic". In universal aging, similar changes occur in all older people as the result of alterations in activation/deactivation of genes that change from a vibrant youthful pattern to a less efficient and effective senescent pattern. For example, reduction in the rate of cell division of senescent gum fibroblasts results in receding gums (Kirkwood and Ritter, 1997). In probabilistic aging, changes may happen to some individuals, not all. For example, in type 2 diabetes, there is age-associated insulin resistance manifested by decreased whole-body tissue sensitivity to insulin (Amati et al., 2009).

Aging is the major risk factor for some neurodegenerative diseases such as Alzheimer's (AD) and Parkinson's (PD) diseases (Ramassamy, 2006). Sporadic PD is a primarily occurring neurodegenerative disorder of advanced ages that affecting about 1% of people over the age of 65 years (Andressoo and Saarma, 2008). The disease is characterized clinically by bradykinesia, tremors at rest, rigidity, disturbance in posture and gait and some neuropsychological deficits (Paulus and Jellinger, 1991). Moreover, neuropsychological deficits, particularly depression and cognitive impairment, have a major negative impact on quality of life in PD (Rahman et al., 2008). Pathologically, the disease is characterized by loss of dopaminergic neurons in substantia nigra (SN) and presence of Lewy bodies in the remaining neurons (Paulus and Jellinger, 1991).

AD is an irreversible progressive brain disorder affecting more than 37 million people over 60 years worldwide. The disease leads to changes in personality, loss of memory and intellectual slowing; moreover, it is the most common cause of dementia in elderly people. The economic burden of AD is massive: for example in the United State alone, the estimated direct and indirect annual cost of patient care is at least US$100 billion (Rafii and Aisen, 2009). There is compelling evidence that acetylcholine-releasing neurons in the basal forebrain selectively degenerate in AD. These cholinergic neurons provide widespread innervations of the cerebral cortex and related structures, and appear to play an important role in cognitive functions, especially memory (Coyle et al., 1983).

Traditional Chinese Medicine (TCM) is a range of traditional medical practices originating in China. TCM is considered an alternative medical system in much of the Western World. TCM practices include herbal medicine, acupuncture, dietary therapy and both *Tui na* and *Shiatsu* massage. More than 2000–3000 years ago, TCM was used by Chinese communities to maintain good health and also to treat diseases (Chan, 2005). In recent years, the use of TCM by other Western countries has been increased and some in the west have begun to recognize TCM as a potential source of new drug candidates (Corson and Crews, 2007; Efferth *et al.*, 2007; Schmidt *et al.*, 2007; Li and Zhang, 2008). Among TCM, Chinese herbal medicine is a major aspect and includes a large number of Chinese herbs that are used by Chinese people for thousands of years to maintain health and treat many disease conditions.

This chapter will address and discuss the role of Chinese herbal medicine in controlling and treating age-related neurodegenerative diseases with special references to PD and AD.

7.2 Role of Chinese Herbal Medicine in Age-Related Neurodegenerative Diseases

Much of growing studies have indicated that a range of Chinese herbs such as *Ginkgo biloba,* green tea, *Panax ginseng, Polygonum multiforum, Tripterygium wilfordii, Nerium indicum, Ganoderma lucidum, Huperzia serrata and Stephania intermedia* have shown potential neuroprotective effects against some of age-related neurodegenerative diseases (Chen *et al.*, 2007). Presence of multiple crude herb materials with many biologically active components in Chinese herbal formulations significantly characterizes them in treating age-related neurodegenerative diseases which have multiple underlying disease mechanisms (Wang *et al.*, 2008).

7.2.1 *Ginkgo biloba*

Ginkgo biloba L. (Ginkgoaceae), *Yin Xing* in Chinese, is one of the oldest living tree species originated from China. Its earliest leaf fossils are dating back to 290 million years ago in the Permian period. It is first introduced

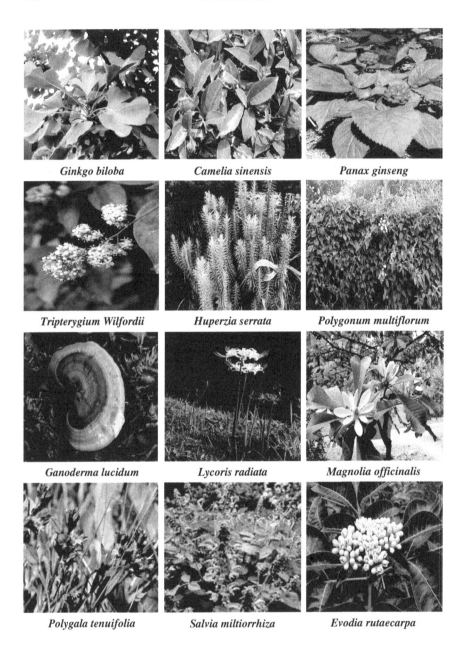

Ginkgo biloba Camelia sinensis Panax ginseng

Tripterygium Wilfordii Huperzia serrata Polygonum multiflorum

Ganoderma lucidum Lycoris radiata Magnolia officinalis

Polygala tenuifolia Salvia miltiorrhiza Evodia rutaecarpa

to Europe in the 18th century. Nowadays, ginkgo supplements are the best-selling herbal medications in Europe and United States and rank as a top medicine prescribed in France and Germany. Ginkgo leaf extract is termed as EGB761 and contains flavonol glycosides (24%), terpene trilactones (6%), proanthoc yanidins (7%) and some other constituents (De Feudis, 1991).

7.2.1.1. *Parkinson's disease*

The beneficial effect of *Ginkgo biloba* extract, EGb761, against PD has been observed in a number of *in vitro* and *in vivo* PD models. In *in vitro* models, Yang *et al.* (2001) found that EGb761 prevented 1-methyl-4-phenylpyridinium (MPP$^+$)-induced apoptosis in pheochromocytoma (PC12) cells. Also, EGb761 was reported to increase cell viability, reduce lactate dehydrogenase (LDH) release, increase Bcl-2 expression and decrease caspases activities in paraquat-treated PC12 cells (Kang *et al.*, 2007). In *in vivo* models, Yang *et al.* (2001) and Kim *et al.* (2004) reported that EGb 761 reduced the behavioral deficits induced by 1-methyl-4-phenyl-1,2,3,6-tetrahydropyridine (MPTP) and 6-OHDA in rats, respectively. Lu *et al.* (2006) found that EGb 761 decreased Bax/Bcl-2 ratios in both young and aged mice. Wu and Zhu (1999) and Rojas *et al.* (2008) demonstrated that EGb 761 significantly attenuated MPTP-induced loss of striatal dopamine levels and loss of tyrosine hydroxylase (TH) immunostaining in the striatum and SN and improved MPTP-induced impairment of locomotion in mice. This neuroprotective effect of EGb 761 is involved inhibition of monamine oxidase (MAO) with subsequent decrease of MPP$^+$ uptake, blockade of lipid peroxidation and reduction of superoxide radical production. Cao *et al.* (2003) observed that EGb decreased levodopa toxicity in rats.

7.2.1.2. *Alzheimer's disease*

There is growing evidence in the literature demonstrating the beneficial effect of *Ginkgo biloba* extract against AD. In *in vitro* models, it was reported that EGb 761 protected hippocampal cells (Howland *et al.*, 1998; Simons *et al.*, 1998) and PC12 cells (Bastianetto *et al.*, 2000;

Yao *et al.*, 2001) against beta amyloid (Aβ) peptide toxicity. These protective effects of EGb 761 against *in vitro* Aβ toxicity could return to its antioxidative, anti-amyloidogenic and anti-apoptotic properties (Ramassamy, 2006). In this context, Ramassamy (2006) found that EGb 761 reduced the level of hydrogen peroxide in neuroblastoma cell lines stably expressing SwAPP695/PSI mutations. Moreover, Smith and Luo (2004) reported that EGb 761 possessed antioxidant and free radical-scavenging activities that is mediating the antiapoptotic machinery and inhibiting amyloid β aggregation. In animal models for AD, Colciaghi *et al.* (2004) found that EGb 761 enhanced spatial learning and memory in transgenic 2576 mice comparable to wild type mice. This beneficial effect of EGb 761 was mediated by attenuating Aβ aggregation (Luo *et al.*, 2002; Yao *et al.*, 2001) and Aβ induced oxidative stress (Smith and Luo, 2003). Moreover, EGb 761 influenced mRNA and protein expression of genes encoding for proteins involved in the pathogenesis of AD (Yao *et al.*, 2004). Clinically, some studies have shown that *Ginkgo biloba* extract exhibited therapeutic activity in a variety of disorders including AD (Mckenna *et al.*, 2001). For instance, it was reported that EGb 761 can improve the cognitive function (Kanowski and Hoerr, 2003; Sierpina *et al.*, 2003), memory (Kanowski *et al.*, 1996) and concentration in patients with AD. Moreover, Rouse (1998) found that EGb 761 was safe and appeared capable of stabilizing and in a substantial number of cases, improving the cognitive performance and the social functioning of demented patients. Hofferberth (1994) and Maurer *et al.* (1997) showed that EGb 761 was helpful for people in early stages of AD as well as for those experiencing another form of dementia. Mazza *et al.* (2006) reported that EGb 761 was found to be nearly as effective against AD as donepezil, a prescription drug used to treat the condition. Puglieli *et al.* (2003) returned these clinical effects to the influence of EGb 761 on the production of brain amyloid precursor protein (APP) and the Aβ peptide by lowering the levels of circulating free cholesterol (Yao *et al.*, 2004) as high cholesterol level could affect the generation and processing of APP.

7.2.2 Green tea

Camelia sinensis L. (Theaceae), *Lu Cha* in Chinese, is the first discovered and recorded tea plant. It has been used to produce tea for about three thousand years. It is native to Southeast Asia and today, it is cultivated across the world in tropical and subtropical regions. Green tea, oolong and black tea, are all harvested from this species depending upon different levels of fermentation, of which green tea (GT) is one of the most popular beverages in the world. GT contains many polyphenol compounds generally known as catechins. The main catechins in GT are epicatechin (EC), epicatechin gallate (ECG), epigallocatechin (EGC) and epigallocatechin gallate (EGCG). Among them, EGCG is the most active and major polyphenol and primarily responsible for the effects of GT (Stewart *et al.*, 2005). GT polyphenols can be absorbed from the digestive tract and high levels of bioavailable GT polyphenols may be detected in the brain (Suganuma *et al.*, 1998). Most of EGCG's effects were reported to return to its powerful antioxidant properties either by direct scavenging free radicals (Qiong *et al.*, 1996) or by indirect increase of endogenous antioxidants (Skrzydlewska *et al.*, 2002).

7.2.2.1 *Parkinson's disease*

Regarding PD, EGCG has been shown to exert neuroprotective/ neurorescue activities in a wide range of cellular and animal models (Mandel *et al.*, 2008). For instance, Zhao (2009) stated that green tea polyphenols protected PC12 and SH-SY5Y cells against 6-OHDA-induced cell death. Our Neurochemical Group, University of Veterinary Medicine, Vienna, have found that EGCG provided some protection against rotenone toxicity in striatal slices in the form of decreasing cellular damages and production of NO˙ radical (Fig. 1, unpublished data). In animal models, EGCG showed neuroprotective activities against MPTP (Levites *et al.*, 2001) and 6-OHDA (Guo *et al.*, 2007) in mice and rats, respectively. These beneficial effects of green tea polyphenols are attributed to a number of mechanisms. For example, Zhao *et al.* (2001) reported that green tea polyphenols served as a powerful antioxidant against free radicals such as superoxide anion, lipid free radicals and hydroxyl radicals. Zhao (2009) mentioned that green tea polyphenols protected against apoptosis through inhibiting expression of Bax, Bad and Mdm2 and upregulating of Bcl-2, Bcl-w and Bcl-xL, prevented the decrease in mitochondrial membrane potential and suppressed

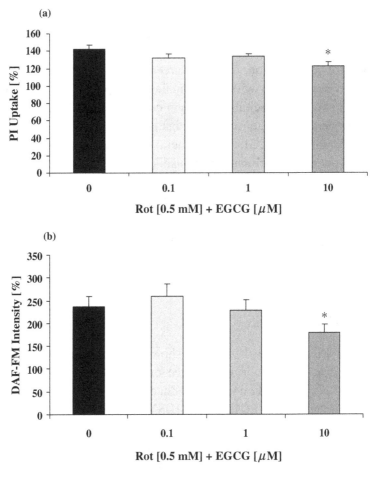

Fig. 7.1. (a) EGCG decreased propidium iodide uptake by strital slices when concomitantly added with rotenone (from day 0 for 48 h). 100% corresponds to the propidium iodide uptake by untreated control slices. Values represent the mean ± SEM of three independent experiments (12–17 slices). Fluorescence intensity was determined densitometrically from ten randomly selected micrographs. (*$p < 0.01$) (b) EGCG decreased NO· production when concomitantly added with rotenone (from day 0 for 48 h). 100% corresponds to the DAF-FM fluorescence intensity in untreated control slices. Values represent the mean ± SEM of three independent experiments (12–17 slices). Fluorescence intensity was determined densitometrically from ten randomly selected micrographs. (*$p < 0.05$).

accumulation of intracellular free calcium. Moreover, green tea polyphenols were reported to decrease NO formation and overexpression of nNOS and iNOS (Guo *et al.*, 2005), inhibited translocation and binding activity of NF-κB and reduced PKC and extracellular signal-regulated kinases (ERK1/2) (Levites *et al.*, 2002a; Levites *et al.*, 2002b). Potent iron-chelating activities also play a role in the neuroprotective activities of green tea polyphenols (Baum and Ng, 2004).

7.2.2.2 *Alzheimer's disease*

Recent research shows that green tea may offer protection against AD through decreasing production of the Alzheimer's-related protein and Aβ which can accumulate abnormally in the brain and lead to nerve damage and memory loss. For instance, Rezai-Zadeh *et al.* (2008) found that EGCG reduced Aβ generation in both murine neuron-like cells (N2a) transfected with the Swedish mutant APP and in primary neurons derived from Swedish mutant APP-overexpressing mice. Lu *et al.* (2006) reported that green tea polyphenols improved animal's learning and memory in AD-like mice induced by D-galactase and Aβ 25–35. This protective effect of green tea polyphenols could be mediated by regulation of the proteolytic processing of the APP and reduction the formation of β-fibrils (Levites *et al.*, 2003).

7.2.3 *Panax ginseng*

Panax ginseng (C.A. MEYER Araliaceae), *renshen* in Chinese, is the most widely used ginseng among the 11th species within the genus Panax. It is a slow-growing perennial plant with fleshly roots in the Northern Hemisphere in eastern Asia (mostly northern China, Korea and eastern Siberia). *Panax ginseng* was first cultivated around 11 BC and has a medical history of more than five thousand years. Today, *Panax ginseng* still occupies a permanent and prominent position in the herbal (best-sellers) list and is considered the most widely herbal product in the world (Blumenthal, 2001). Most of ginseng actions are believed to return to ginsenosides, the principal active ingredients within the roots of *Panax ginseng* (Attele, 1999). Ginsenosides exist in minute amounts in Panax species and it is suggested that each ginsenoside may have its own specific tissue-dependent effects (Murphy and Lee, 2002).

Ginseng products are usually used as a general tonic and adaptogen to help the body to resist the adverse influences of a wide range of physical, chemical and biological factors and to restore homeostasis (Nocerino et al., 2007). Recently, a number of studies described the beneficial effect of ginseng and its main components, ginsenosides, on some neurodegenerative diseases including PD and AD (Van Kampen et al., 2003).

7.2.3.1 *Parkinson's disease*

Growing studies have indicated that ginsenosides, the active ingredients of Panax ginseng, showed neuroprotective effects in PD models. In *in vitro* models, Tohda et al. (2002) reported that the ginseng saponins, Rb1 and Rb3, enhanced the neurite growth of dopaminergic SK-N-SH neuroblastoma cells. Radad et al. (2002a; 2002b) also found that ginsenosides Rb1 and Rg1 increased the survival of dopaminergic neurons and promoted their neuritic growth after exposure of primary mesencephalic cell culture to either MPP^+ or glutamate. In *in vivo* models, the ginsenoside Rg1 was found to increase the number of dopamine neurons in the SN and dopamine levels in the striatum in MPTP-treated mice (Wang et al., 2009) and 6-OHDA-treated rats (Xu et al., 2008). Moreover, Van Kampen et al. (2003) reported that oral administration of ginseng extract G115 decreased the loss of dopamine neurons in SN, diminished the reduction of TH immunoreactivivty in the striatum and preserved striatal dopamine transporter in MPP^+-exposed rats.

The processes and mechanisms underlying the neuroprotective effects of ginseng include (1) suppression of oxidative stress and apoptosis, (2) attenuation of neuroinflammation, (3) potentiation of nerve growth factor, and (4) reduction of nigral iron levels. In parallel, Chun et al. (2003) reported that ginsenoside Rg1 was shown to interrupt dopamine-reduced elevation of reactive oxygen species (ROS) or NO generation in PC12 cells. Kim et al. (2003) and Chen et al. (2002) found that Ginseng radix attenuated MPP^+-induced apoptosis through enhancement of the expression of Bcl-2 and Bcl-xl, reduced expression of Bax and nitric oxide synthase and inhibited activation of caspase-3. Lin et al. (2007) reported that ginsenoside Rd counteracted lipopolysaccharides (LPS)-induced dopaminergic cell loss in primary cell culture through reducing NO formation and PGE2 synthesis. Salim *et al.* (1997) showed that ginsenosides Rb1 and Rg1 elevated mNGF expression in rat brain and Rudakewish *et al.* (2001) concluded that ginsenosides Rb1 and Rg1 potentiated NGF-induced neurite outgrowth in cell culture. Wang *et al.* (2009) reported that ginsenoside Rg1 could reduce nigral iron levels through decreasing the DMT1 expression (iron transporter protein) and FP1 (iron export protein) in SN of MPTP-treated mice.

7.2.3.2 *Alzheimer's disease*

Ginseng is recently found to produce protective and trophic effects against AD. Yang *et al.* (2009) reported that ginsenoside Rg3 significantly reduced the level of $A\beta$ peptide 40 and 42 in SK-N-SH cells transfected with Swedish mutant SweApp through enhancing neprilysin (NEP), the rate-limiting enzyme in the $A\beta$ degradation in the brain. By the way, accumulation of $A\beta$ in the brain is a triggering event leading to the pathological cascade of AD. Moreover, Shieh *et al.* (2008) found that ginsenoside Rh2 could protect type I rat brain astrocytes from apoptosis induced by $A\beta$. This effect of ginsenoside Rh2 is mediated by increasing pituitary adenylate cyclase activating polypeptide (PACAP), a member of the vasoactive intestinal peptide/secretin/glucagen superfamily. In murine models of AD, Zhong *et al.* (2005) reported that *Panax notoginseng* saponins protected cholinergic neurons in rats after intraperitoneal injection of D-galactose combined with NBM injection of the excitatory neurotoxin ibotenic acid. In APP transgenic mice, Cong *et al.* (2007) observed that Naoweikang (NWK), a composite of ginseng and *ginkgo biloba*, increased acetylcholine level which might be one of its mechanisms in improving learning and memory in AD model. Most importantly, ginseng was found to improved cognitive performance in AD patients compared to control group in an open-label study (Lee *et al.*, 2008).

7.2.4 *Tripterygium Wilfordii Hook F (TWHF)*

TWHF (Calastraceae), *Lei Gong Teng* in Chinese, is a deciduous climbing vine growing to 12 meters with brown, angular and downy twigs. The herb comes from the roots, leaves and flowers and used in TCM for treatment of fever, chills, edema and carbuncles. Recently, it has been investigated as a treatment for a variety of disorders including rheumatoid arthritis, chronic hepatitis, chronic nephritis, ankylosing spondylitis as well as several skin diseases. The principal active component of TWHF is triptolide (T_{10}) which is further purified from T_{11}, the active anti-inflammatory components of TWHF. T_{10} was reported to exert anti-inflammatory, immunosuppressive and anti-infertility activities (Zhao et al., 2000). T_{10} can penetrate the blood-brain barrier (BBB) easily because of its lipophilic character and small molecular size (Wang et al., 2008).

7.2.4.1 Parkinson's disease

T_{10}, the most abundant and active ingredient of TWHF, possesses potent neuroprotective properties on dopaminergic neurons both in in vitro and in vivo. In in vitro PD models, Wang et al. (2008) showed that T_{10} can promote the growth of the axons of rat dopaminergic neurons in primary culture and inhibited the cytotoxic effects of MPP on PC12 cells. In in vivo models, it was reported that T_{10} significantly improved the behavior of PD rats, decreased the death of dopaminergic neurons and increased the level of dopamine in the striatum after injection of lipopolysaccharides in the SN (Zhou et al., 2005). Also, T_{10} was found to improve the level of dopamine in the SN and striatum in MPTP-lesioned C57B/6 mice (Hong et al., 2007). The underlying mechanisms that may contribute to the neuroprotective actions of T_{10} include (i) anti-inflammatory effects, (ii) anti-oxidative activities, and (iii) neurotrophins up-regulation. In this context, Li et al. (2004) reported that T_{10} inhibited microglial activation and decreased the release of pro-inflammatory cytokines such as tumor necrosis factor-α (TNF-α) in LPS-treated primary-neuron-glia mixed cultures. He et al. (2003) and Gu et al. (2004) found that T_{10} inhibited the accumulation of ROS induced by glutamate or MPP in PC12 cells. Li et al. (2009) observed that T_{10} improved the expression of brain-derived neurotrophic factor mRNA in primary midbrain cell culture.

7.2.4.2 Alzheimer's disease

T_{10} was found to inhibit apoptosis of PC12 cells induced by Aβ. Gu et al. (2004) attributed these protective effects to the inhibitory effect of T_{10}

on the production of ROS and to recovery the decrease of mitochondrial membrane potential. Moreover, Lee *et al.* (2002) reported that T_{10} inhibited the activation of NF-κB in Aβ-treated PC12 cells.

7.2.5 *Huperzia serrata*

Huperzia serrata Thunb (Lycopodiaceae), *Qian Ceng Ta* in Chinese, is a club moss that has very limited distribution and grows very slowly. It takes at least 15 years from spore germination through the gametophyte stage to finally reach the mature sporophyte stage (Ma *et al.*, 2004). The earliest record of its medicinal usage can be traced back to an ancient Chinese pharmacopeia (Ma *et al.*, 2007). *Huperzia serrata* has become known worldwide as a medicinal plant since Chinese scientists discovered huperzine A in its extract (Ye *et al.*, 2008).

Huperzine A is a natural alkaloid that crosses the BBB smoothly and shows high specify for acetylcholinestrase (AchE) (Wang and Tang, 2005). It was approved as a drug to treat AD in China in 1990s. In this context, it was reported that huperzine A improved learning and memory impairment in a wide range of AD animal models, in elderly people with benign senescent forgetfulness and in patients with AD with minimal peripheral cholinergic side effects and without unexpected toxicity (Zhang *et al.*, 2002; Kuang *et al.*, 2004; Zhang *et al.*, 2008). Moreover, it was shown that huperzine A was eight and two folds more potent than donepezil and rivastigmine, respectively, on cortical acetylcholine levels and AchE activity in rats (Liang and Tang, 2004). The underlying mechanisms that mediate the action of huperzine A beyond the anticholinestrase activity include (1) regulation of APP metabolism, (2) reduction of oxidative stress, (3) protection against apoptosis, and (4) regulation of the expression of nerve growth factor (Zhang and Tang, 2006; Zhang *et al.*, 2008). Respectively, (1) huperzine A was found to direct APP metabolism toward the non-amyloidogenic α-secretase pathway via the mAChR, PKC and MAP kinase pathways in neuroblastoma SK-N-SH APPwt cells (Peng *et al.*, 2007); (2) huperzine A significantly elevated the activities of the antioxidant enzymes such as glutathione perioxidase and catalase, and decreased the level of the lipid peroxidation product malonaldhyde (Xiao *et al.*, 2000); (3) huperzine A protected against Aβ-induced apoptosis in rats through upregulation of the antiapoptotic protein Bcl-2 and down regulation of the pro-apoptotic proteins Bax and p53 (Wang *et al.*, 2001); and (4) huperzine A increased the number of neurite bearing PC12 cells and upregulated the levels of NGFmRNA and P76, the low affinity NGF receptor (Tang *et al.*, 2005). In accordance, these data indicate that huperzine A can be promising for treatment of AD.

7.2.6 *Polygonum multiflorum*

Polygonum multiforum Thunb (Polygonaceae) is a quickly spreading vine that appears in fall, has delicate flowers and covers anything rapidly. It is a widely used Chinese herb to rejuvenate human body. *Polygonum multiforum* Thunb has long been used as a constituent of traditional Chinese prescriptions for treatment of age-related diseases such as cognitive impairment and PD. Li *et al.* (2005) reported that chronic administration of the extract of *Polygonum multiforum* Thunb attenuated the behavioral deficits such as bradykinesia and the degeneration of nigrostriatal dopamine neurons induced by a combination of parquat and maneb in male C57BL/6 mice. The author returned these protective effects to the reduction of oxygen free radicals, inhibition of monoamine oxidase activity, increasing the synaptic dopamine level in the striatum and attenuating the function of cholinergic neurons in the striatum, which counteracts the activity of the striatal dopaminergic system.

Regarding AD, Wang *et al.* (2007) stated that 2, 3, 5, 4`-tetrahydroxystilbene-2-O-beta-d-glucose (TSG), the major component of *Polygonum multiforum* Thunb, may be beneficial for the treatment of AD and the improvement of cognitive impairment in old people. In this context, Wang and his colleagues (2007) found that TSG improved learning-memory abilities, increased the number of synapses and synaptic vesicles and elevated the expression of synaptophysin in the hippocampus when administered orally to 21-month-old rats for three months. Zhang *et al.* (2006) reported that TSG can reserve the learning-memory deficit in the late stage of AD-like model, the PDAPPV7171 transgenic mice. Moreover, Li *et al.* (2003) observed that *Polygonum multiforum* Thunb increased the projecting AchE fibers to the cortex and the hippocampus following treatment with the neurotoxin kainic acid in rats.

7.3 Other Chinese Herbs

7.3.1 *Ganoderma lucidum*

Ganoderma lucidum P. Karst (Ganodermataceae) is one of the oldest mushrooms known to have been used in medicine. It has been used in TCM for more than 4000 years to promote health and increase longevity.

The oil from the spores of *Ganoderma lucidum* was found to improve the behavioral deficits, increase the level of dopamine and DOPAC in the striatum and increase the surviving dopamine neurons in the SN in MPTP-treated mice (Zhu *et al.*, 2005).

Also, the aqueous extract of *Ganoderma lucidum* was found to attenuate Aβ-induced synaptotoxicity by preserving the synaptic density protein and synaptophysin through inhibiting of phosphorylation of c-Jun N-terminal kinase and P38 MAP kinase in cortical neurons (Lai *et al.*, 2008).

7.3.2 *Stephania intermedia*

Stephania intermedia Lo (Menispermaceae) is a flowering plant and is native to eastern and southern Asia. The plant is used in TCM with great caution as it contains toxic amounts of aristolochic acid which can cause renal failure and even death.

Stepholidine (SPD) is an active ingredient of *Stephania intermedia*. SPD can bind to the dopamine D1- and D2-like receptors (Ellenbroek *et al.*, 2006) exhibiting D1 receptor agonistic and D2 receptor antogonisitic activities (Mo *et al.*, 2007). These characters make stepholidine a potential agent in the treatment of drug addiction, PD and particularly, schizophrenia.

Regarding PD, it was reported that SPD may be able to exert symptomatic therapeutic effects and prevent further dopamine neuron degeneration in PD. Li *et al.* (1999) found that SPD protected DA neurons against damage induced by MPTP and MPP$^+$ in rats and can alleviate, in combination with a low dose of bromocriptine, the symptoms of PD in preliminarily clinical trials. Moreover, Yang *et al.* (2007) reported that SPD also relieves the motor PD symptoms when co-administered with Levodopa.

7.3.3 Lycoris radiata Herb

Two alkaloids were isolated from the Chinese herb *Lycoris radiata* Herb (Liliaceae), galantamine and lycoramine. Among them, galantamine was reported to have a powerful selective inhibitory effect on AchE and to stimulate nicotinic receptors (Howes and Houghton, 2003). Therefore, galantamine is licensed in Europe for treatment of AD. Wilcock *et al.* (2000) and Wilkinson and Murray (2001) reported that galantamine improved cognitive function and memory when administered to AD patients in multicentre randomized controlled trials.

7.3.4 Magnolia officinalis

The bark of the root and stem of *Magnolia officinalis* Rehder & Wilson (Magnoliaceae) has been used in TCM to treat anxiety and nervous disturbances. Honokiol and magnolol, two biphenolic lignans isolated from Magnolia officinalis, apparently have multiple actions appropriate for AD therapy. In this context, Hou *et al.* (2000) reported that honokiol and magnolol inhibited AchE activity *in vitro* and increased hippocampal Ach release *in vivo*. Zhou and Xu (1992) and Chen *et al.* (2001) found that the two extracts had antioxidant activity. Lee *et al.* (1998) and Wang *et al.* (1995) reported that magnolol was neuroprotective against chemical hypoxic damage and necrotic cell death in cortical neuron-astrocyte cultures *in vitro* and showed anti-inflammatory activity *in vitro* and *in vivo* perhaps via inhibition of COX and 5-LOX.

7.3.5 Polygala tenuifolia

Polygala tenuifolia Willd (Polygalaceae), *Yuan Zhi* in Chinese, root is firstly used in TCM as a cardiotonic and cerebrotonic, sedative and tranquillizer and for amnesia, neuritis and insomnia (Chang and But, 2001). *Polygala tenuifolia*, with *Panax ginseng*, *Acorus gramineus* and *Poria cocos*, compose a traditional Chinese prescription called DX-9368. DX-9368 showed favorable effects in relation to AD symptoms in several animal models. For example, Zhang *et al.* (1994b) reported that DX-9386 improved memory impairment in mice. Moreover, *Polygala tenuifolia* root extract alone was reported to reserve scopolamine-induced cognitive impairment in rats and protect against glutamate and toxic metabolites of APP *in vitro* (Park *et al.*, 2002). *Polygala tenuifolia* root may also involve anti-inflammatory activity in CNS disorders. For instance, Kim *et al.* (1998) and Koo *et al.* (2000) found that an aqueous extract of *Polygala tenuifolia* root inhibited interleukin-1 mediated TNF secretion by astrocytes and dose-dependently inhibited ethanol-induced interleukin-1 secretion *in vitro*, respectively.

7.3.6 *Salvia miltiorrhiza Bunge*

Salvia miltiorrhiza Bunge (Labiatae), *Tan Shen* in Chinese, is a perennial flowering plant that highly valued for its roots in TCM. The dried root of *Salvia miltiorhiza* is called "Dan shen" in China and has been used for the treatment of CNS deterioration in old age for over one thousand years (Ren *et al.*, 2004). Recently, cryptotanshinone, an active component Saliva miltiorrhiza was seen to strongly attenuate amyloid plaque deposition in the brain of APP/PS1 mice and significantly improved spatial learning and memory in APP/PS1 mice (Mei *et al.*, 2009). The authors attributed these effects of cryptotanshinone to decreasing $A\beta$ generation and promoting APP metabolism toward the non-amyloidogenic products pathway.

7.3.7 *Biota orientalis*

Biota orientalis L. (Coniferae), *Bai Zi Ren* in Chinese, is used in TCM for insomnia and amnesia. S-113m, an herbal prescription is composed of *Biota orientalis*, *Panax ginseng* and *Schisandra chinensis*, was found to improve memory registration and consolidation in mice (Nishiyama *et al.*, 1995a). Also, the seed extract of *Biota orientalis* ameliorated the memory-acquisition disorders induced by amygdala and basal forebrain lesions in mice (Nishiyama *et al.*, 1992; 1995b).

7.3.8 *Coptis chinensis*

Coptis chinensis Franch (Ranunculaceae), *Huang Lian* in Chinese, and some isolated alkaloids (berberine, coptisine and palmatine) were reported to inhibit AchE (Shigeta *et al.*, 2002) and improve a scopolamine-induced learning and memory deficit in rats (Hsieh *et al.*, 2000). Moreover, Shigeta *et al.* (2002) reported that berberine, coptisine and palmatine showed NGF-enhancing activity in PC12 cells.

7.3.9 *Evodia rutaecarpa*

Evodia rutaecarpa Juss. (Rutaceae), *Wu Chu Yu* in Chinese, a Chinese herb used in TCM for cardiotonic, restorative and analgesic effects, was reported to have some pharmacological activities relevant to AD. Park *et al.* (1996) found that *Evodia rutaecarpa* and dehydroevodiamine inhibited AChE *in vitro* and reversed scopolamine-induced memory impairment in rats.

7.3.10 *Nerium indicum*

Nerium indicum Mill. (Apocynaceae) was considered to be an own species for a long time but recently it is regarded as a variety of *Nerium oleander*. The oleander plant grows natively in broad areas from the Mediterranean region trough India to the southern parts of China. Oleander is known to be highly toxic (Langford and Boor, 1996). Ingestion of 15–20 g of fresh leaves might lead to death.

To date, there are no proven benefits of *Nerium indicum*. Nevertheless, some few *in vitro* studies have been indicated putative beneficial effects of plant compounds. Polysaccharides, rhamnogalacturonan and xyloglucan, were extracted from the flowers by Ding *et al.* (2003) and administered on PC 12 cells. Results showed an induction of proliferation and differentiation in PC12 cells. Yu *et al.* (2004) reported neuroprotective effects of polysaccharides, named J2, J3 and J4, from the flowers against serum-deprivation and Aβ peptide toxicity in primary rat cortical neuronal cultures. A decrease of the activity of caspase-3 triggered by Aβ peptides could be observed and an activation of Akt survival signaling pathway. Yu *et al.* (2007) presented a study in which a newly isolated polysaccharide, J6, was used in cultured cortical neurons. This compound markedly inhibited the Aβ peptide-stimulated phosphorylation of JNK-1. Their results pointed to a putative use of *Nerium indicum* polysaccharides as a neuroprotective compound against neuronal death in Alzheimer's disease.

7.4 Concluding Remarks

Chinese herbal medicine is developed as a part of Chinese culture a long time ago to maintain health and keep homeostasis and nowadays, it is recognized as a potential source of new drug candidates. The long history of the use of traditional Chinese herbal medicine, evidences of their benefits against many disease processes, both *in vivo* and *in vitro* studies, and absence of criticizing reports against their use, make the majority of these herbal preparations safe and popular worldwide. Moreover, Chinese herbal preparations would be beneficial against diseases that have multiple underlying mechanisms as they contain many active ingredients. Each active principal could act against one diseases process. However, much research is needed to refine many of these herbal preparations for specific types of infections, illnesses and diseases and also to avoid their negative interactions with medicines, foods and supplements.

References

Amati, F., Dubé, J.J., Coen, P.M., Stefanovic-Racic, M., Toledo, F.G. and Goodpaster, B.H. (2009) Physical Inactivity and Obesity Underlie the Insulin Resistance of Aging. *Diabetes Care* **32**(8), 1547–1549.

Andressoo, J.O. and Saarma, M. (2008) Signalling mechanisms underlying development and maintenance of dopamine neurons. *Curr. Opin. Neurobiol.* **18**, 297–306.

Attele, A.S., Wu, J.A. and Yuan, C.S. Ginseng pharmacology: Multiple constituents and multiple actions. *Biochem. Pahrmacol.* **58**, 1685–1693.

Bastianetto, S., Ramassamy, C., Dore, S., Christen, Y., Poirier, J. and Quirion R. (2000) The *Ginkgo biloba* extract (EGb 761) protects hippocampal neurons against cell death induced by beta-amyloid. *Eur. J. Neurosci.* **12**, 1882–1890.

Baum, L. and Ng, A. (2004) Curcumin interaction with copper and iron suggests one possible mechanism of action in Alzheimer's disease animal models. *J. Alzheimers. Dis.* **6**, 367–377.

Blumenthal, M. (2001) Asian ginseng: Potential therapeutic uses. *Adv. Nurse. Pract.* **2**, 26–28.

Cao, F., Sun, S. and Tong, E.T. (2003) Experimental study on inhibition of neuronal toxical effect of levodopa by *Ginkgo biloba* extract on Parkinson disease in rats. *J. Huazhong Univ. Sci. Tech. Med. Sci.* **23**, 151–153.

Chan, K. (2005) Chinese medicinal materials and their interface with Western medical concepts. *J. Ethnopharmacol.* **96**, 1–18.

Chang, H. and But, P.P. (2001) *Pharmacology and Applications of Chinese Material Medica*, Vol. 1–2. World Scientific Singapore.

Chen, L.W., Wang, Y.Q., Wei, L.C., Shi, M. and Chan, Y.S. (2007) Chinese herbs and herbal extracts for neuroprotection of dopaminergic neurons and potential therapeutic treatment of Parkinson's disease. *CNS Neurol. Disord. Dr.* **6**, 273–281.

Chen, X.C., Chen, Y., Zhu, Y.G., Fang, F. and Chen, L.M. (2002) Protective effect of ginsenoside Rg1 against MPTP-induced apoptosis in mouse substantia nigra neurons. *Acta Pharmacol. Sin.* **23**, 829–834.

Chen, Y.L., Lin, K.F., Shiao, M.S., Chen, Y.T., Hong, C.Y. and Lin, S.J. (2001) Magnolol, a potent antioxidant from *Magnolia officinalis*, attenuates intimal thickening and MCP-1 expression after balloon injury of the aorta in cholesterol-fed rabbits. *Basic Res. Cardiol.* **96**, 353–363.

Chun, C.X., Gui, Z.Y., An, Z.L., Chun, H., Ying, C. and Min C.L. (2003) Ginsenoside Rg1 attenuates dopamine-induced apoptosis in PC12 cells by suppressing oxidative stress. *Eur. J. Pharmacol.* **473**,1–7.

Colciaghi, F., Borroni, B., Zimmermann, M., Bellone, C., Longhi, A., Padovani, A., Cattabeni, F., Christen, Y. and Di Luca, M. (2004) Amyloid precursor protein metabolism is regulated toward alpha-secretase pathway by *Ginkgo biloba* extracts. *Neurobiol. Dis.* **16**, 454–460.

Cong, W.H., Liu, J.X. and Xu, L. Effects of extracts of Ginseng and *Ginkgo biloba* on hippocampal acetylcholine and monoamines in PDAP-pV717I transgenic mice. *Zhongguo Zhong Xi Yi Jie He Za Zhi* **27**, 810–813.

Corson, T.W. and Crews, C.M. (2007) Molecular understanding and modern application of traditional medicines: Triumphs and trials. *Cell* **130**, 769–774.

Coyle, J.T., Price, D.L. and DeLong, M.R. (1983) Alzheimer's disease: A disorder of cortical cholinergic innervation. *Science* **219**, 1184–1190.

De Feudis, F.V. (1991) *Ginkgo Biloba Extract EGb 761: Pharmacological Activities and Clinical Applications*. Elsevier, Paris, pp. 1–8.

Ding, K., Fang, J.N., Dong, T., Tsim, K.W. and Wu, H. (2003) Characterization of a rhamnogalacturonan and a xyloglucan from neriumindicum and their activities on PC12 pheochromocytoma cells. *Nat. Prod.* **66**, 7–10.

Efferth, T., Li, P.C.H., Konkimalla, V.S.B. and Kaina, B. (2007) From traditional Chinese medicine to rational cancer therapy. *Trends Mol. Med.* **13**, 353–361.

Ellenbroek, B.A., Zhang, X.X. and Jin, G.Z. Effects of (–)stepholidine in animal models for schizophrenia. *Acta Pharmacol. Sin.* **27**, 1111–1118.

Gu, M., Zhou, H.F., Xue, B., Niu, D.B. and Wang, X.M. (2004) The effect of chinese herb *Tripterygium wilfordii* Hook F. monomer T_{10} on *in vitro* model of Alzheimer's disease. *Acta Physiol. Sin.* **56**, 73–78.

Guo, S., Yan, J., Bezard, E., Yang, T., Yang, X. and Zhao B. (2007) Protective effects of green tea polyphenols in the 6-OHDA rat model of Parkinson's disease through inhibition of ROS-NO pathway. *Biol. Psychiat.* **62**, 1353–1362.

Guo, S.H., Bezard, E. and Zhao, B.L. (2005) Protective effect of green tea polyphenols on the SH-SY5Y cells against 6-OHDA induced apoptosis through ROS-NO pathway. *Free Radic. Biol. Med.* **39**, 682–695.

He, Q.H., Zhou, H.F., Xue, B., Niu, D.B. and Wang, X.M. Neuroprotective effects and mechanism of *Tripteryygium wilforddi* Hook F monomer triptolide on glutamate induced PC12 cell line damage. *Beijing Da Xue Xue Bao* **35**, 252–255.

Hofferberth, B. (1994) The efficacy of EGb 761 in patients with senile dementia of the Alzheimers type, a double-blind, placebo-controlled study on different levels of investigation. *Hum. Psychopharmacol.* **9**, 215–222.

Hong, Z., Wang, G., Gu, J., Pan, J., Bai, L., Zhang, S. and Chen, S.D. (2007) Tripchlorolide protects against MPTP-induced neurotoxicity in C57BL/6 mice. *Eur. J. Neurosci.* **26**, 1500–1508.

Hou, Y.C., Chao, P.D. and Chen, S.Y. (2000) Honokiol and magnolol increased hippocampal acetylcholine release in freely-moving rats. *Am. J. Chin. Med.* **28**, 379–384.

Howes, M-J.R. and Houghtonb, P.J. (2003) Plants used in Chinese and Indian traditional medicine for improvement of memory and cognitive function. *Pharmacol. Biochem. Be.* **75**, 513–527.

Howland, D.S., Trusko, S.P., Savage, M.J., Reaume, A.G., Lang, D.M., Hirsch, J.D., Maeda, N., Siman, R., Greenberg, B.D., Scott, R.W. and Flood, D.G. (1998) Modulation of secreted beta-amyloid precursor protein and amyloid beta-peptide in brain by cholesterol. *J. Biol. Chem.* **273**, 16576–16582.

Hsieh, M.T., Peng, W.H., Wu, C.R. and Wang, W.H. (2000) The ameliorating effects of the cognitive-enhancing Chinese herbs on scopolamine-induced amnesia in rats. *Phytother. Res.* **14**, 375–377.

Kang, X., Chen, J., Xu, Z., Li, H. and Wang, B. (2007) Protective effects of *Ginkgo biloba* extract on paraquat-induced apoptosis of PC12 cells. *Toxicol. In Vitro* **21**, 1003–1009.

Kanowski, S. and Hoerr R. (2003) *Ginkgo biloba* extract EGb 761 in dementia: Intent-to-treat analyses of a 24-week, multi-center, double-blind, placebo-controlled, randomized trial. *Pharmacopsychiatry* **36**, 297–303.

Kanowski, S., Herrmann, W.M., Stephan, K., Wierich, W. and Horr R. (1996) Proof of efficacy of the *ginkgo biloba* special extract EGb 761 in outpatients suffering from mild to moderate primary degenerative dementia of the Alzheimer type or multi-infarct dementia. *Pharmacopsychiatry* **29**, 47–56.

Kim, E.H., Jang, M.H., Shin, M.C., Shin, M.S. and Kim, C.J. (2003) Protective effect of aqueous extract of Ginseng radix against 1-methyl-4-phenylpyridinium-induced apoptosis in PC12 cells. *Biol Pharm Bull* **26**, 1668–1673.

Kim, H.M., Lee, E.H., Na, H.J., Lee, S.B., Shin, T.Y., Lyu, Y.S., Kim, N.S. and Nomura S. (1998) Effect of *Polygala tenuifolia* root extract on the tumour necrosis factor-a secretion from mouse astrocytes. *J. Ethnopharmacol.* **61**, 201–208.

Kim, M.S., Leem, J.I., Lee, W.Y. and Kim, S.E. (2004) Neuroprotective effect of *Ginkgo biloba L.* extract in a rat model of Parkinson's disease. *Phytother. Res.* **18**, 663–666.

Kirkwood, T.B. and Ritter, M.A. (1997) The interface between ageing and health in man. *Age Ageing* **4**, 9–14.

Koo, H.N., Jeong, H.J., Kim, K.R., Kim, J.C., Kim, K.S. and Kang, B.K., *et al.* (2000) Inhibitory effect of interleukin-1a-induced apoptosis by *Polygala tenuifolia* in Hep H2 cells. *Immunopharmacol. Immunotoxicol.* **22**(3), 531–544.

Kuang, M.Z., Xiao, W.M., Wang, S.F. and Li, R.X. (2004) Clinical evaluation of huperzine A in improving intelligent disorder in patients with Alzheimer's disease. *Chin.J. Clin. Rehabil.* **8**, 1216–1217.

Lai, C.S., Yu, M.S., Yuen, W.H., So, K.F., Zee, S.Y., Chang, R.C. (2008) Antagonizing beta-amyloid peptide neurotoxicity of the anti-aging fungus *Ganoderma lucidum. Brain Res.* **23**, 215–224.

Langford, S.D. and Boor, P.J. (1996) Oleander toxicity: An examination of human and animal toxic exposures. *Toxicology* **109**, 1–13.

Lee, K.Y., Park, J.S., Jee, Y.K. and Rosen, G.D. (2002) Triptolide sensitizes lung cancer cells to TNF-related apoptosis-inducing ligand (TRAIL)-induced apoptosis by inhibition of NF-kappaB activation. *Exp. Mol. Med.* **34**, 462–468.

Lee, M.M., Hseih, M.T., Kuo, J.S., Yeh, F.T. and Huang, H.M. (1998) Magnolol protects cortical neuronal cells from chemical hypoxia in rats. *Neuroreport* **9**, 3451–3456.

Lee, S.T., Chu, K., Sim, J.Y., Heo, J.H. and Kim, M. (2008) *Panax ginseng* enhances cognitive performance in Alzheimer disease. *Alzheimer Dis. Assoc. Disord.* **22**, 222–226.

Levites, Y., Amit, T., Mandel, S. and Youdim, M.B. (2003) Neuroprotection and neurorescue against Abeta toxicity and PKC-dependent release of nonamyloidogenic soluble precursor protein by green tea polyphenol (−)-epigallocatechin-3-gallate. *FASEB J* **17**, 952–954.

Levites, Y., Amit, T., Youdim, M.B.H. and Mandel S. (2002b) Involvement of protein kinase C activation and cell survival/cell cycle genes in green tea polyphenol-epigallocatechin 3-gallate neuroprotective action. *J. Biol. Chem.* **77**, 30574–30580.

Levites, Y., Weinreb, O., Maor, G., Youdim, M.B.H. and Mandel S. (2001) Green tea polyphenol epigallocatechin-3-gallate prevents MPTP induced dopaminergic neurodegeneration. *J. Neurochem.* **78**, 1073–1082.

Levites, Y., Youdima, M.B.H., Mao, G. and Mandel S. (2002a) Attenuation of 6-OHDA-induced nuclear factor-NF-kB activation and celldeath by tea extracts in neuronal cultures. *Biochem. Pharmacol.* **63**, 21–29.

Li, F.Q., Cheng, X.X., Liang, X.B., Wang, X.H., Bing, X., He, Q.H., Wang, X.M. and Han, J.S. (2003) Neurotrophic and neuroprotective effects of Tripchlorolide, an extract of Chinese herb *Tripterygium wilfordii* Hook F, on dopaminergic neurons. *Exp. Neurol.* **179**, 28–37.

Li, F.Q., Lu, X.Z., Liang, X.B., Zhou, H.F., Xue, B., Liu, X.Y., Niu, D.B., Han, J.S. and Wang, X.M. (2004) Triptolide, a Chinese herbal extract, protects dopaminergic neurons from inflammation-mediated damage through inhibition of microglial activation. *J. Neuroimmunol.* **148**, 24–31.

Li, M., Du, X.P. and Ye, H. (2003) Protective effect of *Polygonum multiflorum* thunb on the cerebral cholinergic neurofibers in rats. *Hunan Yi Ke Da Xue Xue Bao* **28**, 361–364.

Li, P.K., Chen, L.J., Zhao, H. and Jin, G.Z. (1999) Treatment of Parkinson disease with l-stepholidine (SPD) plus bromocriptine. *Chin. J. Integr. Tradit. West. Med.* **19**, 428–429.

Li, X., Matsumoto, K., Murakami, Y., Tezuka, Y., Wu, Y. and Kadota, S. (2005) Neuro-protective effects of *Polygonum multiflorum* on nigrostriatal dopaminergic degeneration induced by paraquat and maneb in mice. *Pharmacol. Biochem. Behav.* **82**, 345–352.

Li, X.-J. and Zhang, H.-Y. (2008) Western-medicine-validated anti-tumor agents and traditional Chinese medicine. *Trends. Mol. Med.* **14**, 1–2.

Liang, Y.Q. and Tang, X.C. (2004) Comparative effects of huperzine A, donepezil and rivastigmine on cortical acetylcholine level and acetylcholinesterase activity in rats. *Neurosci. Lett.* **361**, 56–59.

Lin, W.M., Zhang, Y.M., Moldzio, R. and Rausch, W.D. (2007) Ginsenoside Rd attenuates neuroinflammation of dopaminergic cells in culture. *J. Neural. Transm. Suppl.* **72**, 105–112.

Lu, G., Wu, Y., Mak, Y.T., Wai, S.M., Feng, Z.T., Rudd, J.A. and Yew, D.T. (2006) Molecular evidence of the neuroprotective effect of *Ginkgo biloba* (EGb761) using Bax/Bcl-2 ratio after brain ischemia in senescence-accelerated mice, strain prone-8. *Brain Res.* **1090**, 23–28.

Lü, J.H., Guo, J. and Yang, W.H. (2006) Effects of green tea polyphenol on the behaviour of Alzheimer's disease like mice induced by D-galactose and Abeta25–35. *Zhong Yao Cai* **29**, 352–324.

Luo, Y., Smith, J.V., Paramasivam, V., Burdick, A., Curry, K.J., Buford, J.P., Khan, I., Netzer, W.J., Xu, H. and Butko, P. (2002) Inhibition of amyloid-beta aggregation and caspase-3 activation by the *Ginkgo biloba* extract EGb761. *PNc. Natl. Acad. Sci.* **99**, 12197–12202.

Ma, X. and Gang, D.R. (2007) The Lycopodium alkaloids. *Nat. Prod. Rep.* **21**, 752–772.

Ma, X., Tan, C., Zhu, D., Gang, D.R. and Xiao, P. (2007) Huperzine A from Huperzia species: An ethnopharmacological review. *J. Ethnopharmacol.* **113**, 15–34.

Mandel, S.A., Amit, T., Weinreb, O., Reznichenko, L. and Youdim, M.B. (2008) Simultaneous manipulation of multiple brain targets by green tea catechins: A potential neuroprotective strategy for Alzheimer and Parkinson diseases. *CNS Neurosci. Ther.* **4**, 352–365.

Maurer, K., Ihl, R., Dierks, T. and Frolich, L. (1997) Clinical efficacy of *Ginkgo biloba* special extract EGb 761 in dementia of the Alzheimers type. *J. Psychiatr. Res.* **31**(6), 645–655.

Mazza, M., Capuano, A., Bria, P. and Mazza, S. (2006) *Ginkgo biloba* and donepezil: A comparison in the treatment of Alzheimer's dementia in a randomized placebo-controlled double-blind study. *Eur. J. Neurol.* **13**, 981–985.

McKenna, D.J., Jones, K. and Hughes, K. (2001) Efficacy, safety and use of *ginkgo biloba* in clinical and preclinical applications. *Altern. Ther. Health Med.* **7**, 88–90.

Mei, Z., Zhang, F., Tao, L., Zheng, W., Cao, Y., Wang, Z., Tang, S., Le, K., Chen, S., Pi, R. and Liu, P. (2009) Cryptotanshinone, a compound from *Salvia miltiorrhiza* modulates amyloid precursor protein metabolism and attenuates beta-amyloid deposition through upregulating alpha-secretase *in vivo* and *in vitro*. *Neurosci. Lett.* **452**, 90–95.

Mo, J., Guo, Y., Yang, Y.S., Shen, J.S., Jin, G.Z. and Zhen, X. (2007) Recent developments in studies of l-stepholidine and its analogs: Chemistry, pharmacology and clinical implications. *Curr. Med. Chem.* **14**, 2996–3002.

Murphy, L.L. and Lee, T.J. (2002) Ginseng, sex behavior and nitric oxide. *Ann. NY Acad. Sci.* **962**, 372–377.

Nishiyama, N., Chu, P.J. and Saito, H. (1995b) Beneficial effects of Biota, a traditional Chinese herbal medicine on learning impairment induced by basal forebrain-lesion in mice. *Biol. Pharm. Bull.* 28,1513–1517.

Nishiyama, N., Wang, Y.L and Saito, H. (1995a) Beneficial effects of S-113m, a novel herbal prescription, on learning impairment model in mice. *Biol. Pharm. Bull.* 18,1498–1503.

Nishiyama, N., Yuan-Liang, W., Kaimori, J., Ishihara, A. and Saito H. (1992) Biota (*Po-Tzu Jen*), a traditional Chinese medicine, ameliorates the memory acquisition disorder induced by amygdala lesion in mice. *Phytother. Res.* **6**, 289–293.

Nocerino, E., Amato, M. and Izzo, A.A. (2000) The aphrodisiac and adaptogenic properties of ginseng. *Fitoterapia* **71**, 1–5.

Park, C.H., Choi, S.H., Koo, J.W., Seo, J.H., Kim, H.S., Jeong, S.J. and Suh, Y.H. (2002) Novel cognitive improving and neuroprotective activities of *Polygala tenuifolia* Willldenow extract, BT-11. *J. Neurosci. Res.* **70**, 484–492.

Park, C.H., Kim, S., Choi, W., Lee, Y., Kim, J., Kang, S.S. and Suh, Y.H. (1996) Novel anticholinesterase and antiamnesic activities of dehydroevodiamine, a constituent of *Evodia ruraecarpa*. *Planta Med.* **62**, 405–409.

Paulus, W. and Jellinger, K. (1991) The neuropathologic basis of different clinical subgroups of Parkinson's disease. *J. Neuropathol. Exp. Neurol.* **50**, 743–755.

Peng, Y., Lee, D.Y., Jiang, L., Ma, Z., Schachter, S.C. and Lemere, C.A. Huperzine A regulates amyloid precursor protein processing via protein kinase C and mitogen-activated protein kinase pathways in neuroblastoma SK-N-SH cells over-expressing wild type human amyloid precursor protein 695. *Neuroscience* **150**, 386–395.

Puglielli, L., Tanzi, R.E. and Kovacs, D.M. (2005) Alzheimer's disease: The cholesterol connection. *Nat. Neurosci.* **6**, 345–351.

Qiong, G., Baolu, Z., Meifen, L., Shengrong, S. and Wenjuan, X. (1996) Studies on protective mechanisms of four components of green tea polyphenols against lipid peroxidation in synaptosomes. *Biochim. Biophys. Acta* **1304**, 210–222.

Radad, K., Gille, G., Moldzio, R., Saito H. and Rausch, W.D. (2004a) Ginsenosides Rb1 and Rg1 effects on mesencephalic dopaminergic cells stressed with glutamate. *Brain Res.* **17**, 41–53.

Radad, K., Gille, G., Moldzio, R., Saito, H., Ishige, K. and Rausch, W.D. (2004b) Ginsenosides Rb1 and Rg1 effects on survival and neurite growth of MPP$^+$-affected mesencephalic dopaminergic cells. *J. Neural. Transm.* **111**, 37–45.

Rafii, M.S. and Aisen, P.S. (2009) Recent developments in Alzheimer's disease therapeutics. *BMC Med.* **7**, 7–10.

Rahman, S., Griffin, H.J., Quinn, N.P. and Jahanshahi, M. (2008) Quality of life in Parkinson's disease: The relative importance of the symptoms. *Mov. Disord.* **30**, 1428–1434.

Ramassamy, C. (2006) Emerging role of polyphenolic compounds in the treatment of neurodegenerative diseases: A review of their intracellular targets. *Eur. J. Pharmacol.* **545**, 51–64.

Ren, Y., Houghton, P.J., Hider, R.C. and Howes, M.J. (2004) Novel diterpenoid acetylcholinesterase inhibitors from *Salvia miltiorhiza. Planta Med.* **70**, 201–204.

Rezai-Zadeh, K., Arendash, G.W., Hou, H., Fernandez, F., Jensen, M., Runfeldt, M., Shytle, R.D. and Tan, J. (2008) Green tea epigallocatechin-3-gallate (EGCG) reduces beta-amyloid mediated cognitive impairment and modulates tau pathology in Alzheimer transgenic mice. *Brain Res* **1214**, 177–187.

Rojas, P., Serrano-García, N., Mares-Sámano, J.J., Medina-Campos, O.N., Pedraza-Chaverri, J. and Ogren, S.O. (2008) EGb761 protects against nigrostriatal dopaminergic neurotoxicity in 1-methyl-4-phenyl-1,2,3,6-tetrahydropyridine-induced Parkinsonism in mice: Role of oxidative stress. *Eur. J. Neurosci.* **28**, 41–50.

Rouse, J. (1998) *Ginkgo biloba*: Mind, mood and memory. J. Appl. Nut. Sci. **6**, 1–2.

Rudakewich, M., Ba, F. and Benishin, C.G. (2001) Neurotrophic and neuroprotective actions of ginsenosides Rb1 and Rg1. *Planta Med.* **67**, 533–537.

Salim, K.N., McEven, B.S. and Choa, H.M. Ginsenoside Rb1 regulates ChAT, NGF and trkA mRNA expression in the rat brain. *Brain Res. Mol. Brain. Res.* **47**, 177–182.

Schmidt, B.M., Ribnicky, D.M., Lipsky, P.E. and Raskin, I. (2007) Revisiting the ancient concept of botanical therapeutics. *Nat. Chem. Biol.* **3**, 360–366.

Shieh, P.C., Tsao, C.W., Li, J.S., Wu, H.T., Wen, Y.J, Kou, D.H. and Cheng, J.T. (2008) Role of pituitary adenylate cyclase-activating polypeptide (PACAP) in the action of ginsenoside Rh2 against beta-amyloid-induced inhibition of rat brain astrocytes. *Neurosci. Lett.* **434**, 1–5.

Shigeta, K., Ootaki, K., Tatemoto, H., Nakanishi, T., Inada, A. and Muto, N. (2002) Potentiation of nerve growth factor-induced neurite outgrowth in PC12 cells by a *Coptidis Rhizoma* extract and protoberberine alkaloids. *Biosci. Biotechnol. Biochem.* **66**, 2491–2494.

Sierpina, V.S., Wollschlaeger, B. and Blumenthal, M. (2003) *Ginkgo biloba. Am. Fam. Physician.* **68**, 923–926.

Simons, M., Keller, P., De Strooper, B., Beyreuther, K., Dotti, C.G. and Simons K. (1998) Cholesterol depletion inhibits the generation of beta-amyloid in hippocampal neurons. *Proc. Natl. Acad. Sci.* **95**, 6460–6464.

Skrzydlewska, E., Ostrowska, J., Farbiszewski, R. and Michalak, K. (2002) Protective effect of green tea against lipid peroxidation in the rat liver, blood serum and the brain. *Phytomedicine* **9**, 232–238.

Smith, J.V. and Luo, Y. Studies on molecular mechanisms of *Ginkgo biloba* extract. *Appl. Microbiol. Biotechol.* **64**, 465–472.

Smith, J.V. and Luo, Y.J. Elevation of oxidative free radicals in Alzheimer's disease models can be attenuated by *Ginkgo biloba* extract EGb 761. *J. Alzheimers Dis* **5**(4), 287–300.

Stewart, A.J., Mullen, W. and Crozier, A. (2005) On-line high-performance liquid chromatography analysis of the antioxidant activity of phenolic compounds in green and black tea. *Mol. Nutr. Food. Res.* **49**, 52–60.

Suganuma, M., Okabe, S., Oniyama, M., Tada, Y., Ito, H. and Fujiki H. (1998) Wide distribution of [3H](−)-epigallocatechin gallate, a cancer preventive tea polyphenol, in mouse tissue. *Carcinogenesis* **19**, 1771–1776.

Tang, L.L., Wang, R. and Tang, X.C. (2005) Effects of huperzine A on secretion of nerve growth factor in cultured rat cortical astrocytes and neurite outgrowth in rat PC12 cells. *Acta Pharmacol. Sin.* **26**, 673–678.

Tohda, C., Matsumoto, N., Zou, K., Meselhy, M.R. and Komatsu K. (2002) Axonal and dendritic extension by protopanaxadiol-type saponins from ginseng drugs in SK-N-SH cells. *Jpn. J. Pharmacol.* **90**, 254–262.

Van Kampen, J., Robertson, H., Hagg, T. and Drobitch, R. (2003) Neuroprotective actions of the ginseng extract G115 in two rodent models of Parkinson's disease. *Exp. Neurol.* **184**, 21–29.

Wang, J., Xu, H.M., Yang, H.D., Du, X.X., Jiang, H. and Xie, J.X. (2009) Rg1 reduces nigral iron levels of MPTP-treated C57BL6 mice by regulating certain iron transport proteins. **54**, 43–48.

Wang, J.P., Hsu, M.F., Raung, S.L., Chen. C.C., Kuo, J.S. and Teng, C.M. (1992) Anti-inflammatory and analgesic effects of magnolol. *Naunyn Schmiedebergs Arch Pharmacol.* **346**, 707–712.

Wang, R. and Tang, X.C. (2005) Neuroprotective effects of huperzine A, a natural cholinesterase inhibitor for the treatment of Alzheimer's disease. *Neurosignals* **14**, 71–82.

Wang, R., Tang, Y., Feng, B., Ye, C., Fang, L., Zhang, L. and Li, L. (2007) Changes in hippocampal synapses and learning-memory abilities in age-increasing rats and effects of tetrahydroxystilbene glucoside in aged rats. *Neuroscience* **23**, 739–746.

Wang, R., Zhang, H.Y. and Tang, X.C. (2001) Huperzine A attenuates cognitive dysfunction and neuronal degeneration caused by beta-amyloid protein-(1–40) in rat. *Eur. J. Pharmacol.* **421**, 149–156.

Wang, X., Liang, X.B., Li, F.Q., Zhou, H.F., Liu, X.Y., Wang, J.J. and Wang, X.M. (2008) Therapeutic strategies for Parkinson's Disease: The ancient meets the future — traditional Chinese herbal medicine, electroacupuncture, gene therapy and stem cells. *Neurochem. Res.* **33**, 1956–1963.

Wang, X., Xi-Bin, L., Feng-Qiao, L., Hui-Fang, Z., Xian-Yu, L., Jian-Jun, W. and Xiao-Min, W. (2008) Therapeutic strategies for Parkinson's disease: The ancient meets the future — traditional chinese herbal medicine, electroacupuncture, gene therapy and stem cells. *Neurochem. Res.* **33**, 1956–1963.

Wilcock, G.K., Lilienfeld, S. and Gaens, E., on behalf of the Galantamine International-1 Study Group (2000) Efficacy and safety of galantamine in patients with mild to moderate Alzheimer's disease: Multicentre randomized controlled trial. *Brit. Med. J.* **321**, 1445–1449.

Wilkinson, D. and Murray, J. (2001) Galantamine: A randomised, double-blind, dose comparison in patients with Alzheimer's disease. *Int. J. Geriatr. Psychiat.* **16**, 852–857.

Wu, W.R. and Zhu, X.Z. (1999) Involvement of monoamine oxidase inhibition in neuroprotective and neurorestorative effects of *Ginkgo biloba* extract against MPTP-induced nigrostriatal dopaminergic toxicity in C57 mice. *Life Sci.* **65**, 157–164.

Xiao, X.Q., Wang, R., Han, Y.F. and Tang, X.C. (2000) Protective effects of huperzine A on beta-amyloid(25–35) induced oxidative injury in rat pheochromocytoma cells. *Neurosci. Lett.* **286**, 155–158.

Xu, L., Liu, L.X. and Chen, W.F. (2008) Effect and mechanism of ginsenoside Rg1 on dopamine contents of striatum in rat model of Parkinson's disease. *Zhongguo Zhong Yao Za Zhi* **33**, 1856–1859.

Yang, K., Jin, G. and Wu, J. (2007) The neuropharmacology of (−)-Stepholidine and its potential applications. *Curr. Neuropharm.* **5**, 289–294.

Yang, L., Hao, J., Zhang, J., Xia, W., Dong, X., Hu, X., Kong, F. and Cui, X. (2009) Ginsenoside Rg3 promotes beta-amyloid peptide degradation by enhancing gene expression of neprilysin. *J. Pharm. Pharmacol.* **61**, 375–380.

Yang, S.F., Yang, Z.Q., Wu, Q., Sun, A.S., Huang, X.N. and Shi, J.S. (2001) Protective effect and mechanism of *Ginkgo biloba* leaf extracts for Parkinson disease induced by 1-methyl-4-pheny1-1,2,3,6-tetra-hydropyridine. *Acta Pharmacol. Sin.* **22**, 1089–1093.

Yao, Z., Drieu, K. and Papadopoulos, V. (2001) The *Ginkgo biloba* extract EGb 761 rescues the PC12 neuronal cells from beta-amyloid-induced cell death by inhibiting the formation of beta-amyloid-derived diffusible neurotoxic ligands. *Brain Res.* **889**, 181–190.

Yao, Z.X., Han, Z., Drieu, K. and Papdopoulos, V. (2004) *Ginkgo biloba* extract (Egb 761) inhibits beta-amyloid production by lowering free cholesterol levels. *J. Nutr. Biochem.* **15**, 749–756.

Ye, J.C., Zengb, S., Zheng, G.L. and Chena, G.S. (2008) Pharmacokinetics of Huperzine A after transdermal and oral administration in beagle dogs. *Int.J. Pharm.* **356**, 187–192.

Yu, M.S., Lai, S.W., Lin, K.F., Fang, J.N., Yuen, W.H. and Chang RC. (2004) Characterization of polysaccharides from the flowers of *Nerium indicum* and their neuroprotective effects. *Int. J. Mol. Med.* **14**, 917–924.

Yu, M.S., Wong, A.Y., So, K.F., Fang, J.N., Yuen, W.H. and Chang, R.C. (2007) New polysaccharide from *Nerium indicum* protects neurons via stress kinase signaling pathway. *Brain Res.* **1153**, 221–230.

Youdim, K.A. and Joseph, J.A. (2001) A possible emerging role of phytochemicals in improving age-related neurological dysfunctions: A multiplicity of effects. *Free. Radic. Biol. Med.* **30**, 583–594.

Zhang, H.Y. and Tang, X.C. (2006) Neuroprotective effects of huperzine A: New therapeutic targets for neurodegenerative disease. *Trends Pharmacol. Sci.* **27**, 619–625.

Zhang, H.Y., Zheng, C.Y., Yan, H., Wang, Z.F., Tang, L.L., Gao, X. and Tang, X.C. (2008) Potential therapeutic targets of huperzine A for Alzheimer's disease and vascular dementia. *Chem. Biol. Interact.* **175**, 396–402.

170

Zhang, L., Xing, Y., Ye, C,F., Ai, H.X., Wei, H.F. and Li, L. (2006) Learning-memory deficit with aging in APP transgenic mice of Alzheimer's disease and intervention by using tetrahydroxystilbene glucoside. *Behav. Brain. Res.* **173**, 246–254.

Zhang, Y., Takashina, K., Saito, H. and Nishiyama, N. (1994b) Anti-aging effect of DX-9368 in senescence accelerated mouse. *Biol Pharm Bull* **17**, 866–868.

Zhang, Z., Wang, X., Chen, Q., Shu, L., Wang, J. and Shan, G. (2002) Clinical efficacy and safety of huperzine Alpha in treatment of mild to moderate Alzheimer disease, a placebo-controlled, double-blind, randomized trial. *Zhonghua Yi Xue Za Zhi* **82**, 941–944.

Zhao, B. (2009) Natural antioxidants protect neurons in Alzheimer's disease and Parkinson's disease. *Neurochem. Res.* **34**, 630–638.

Zhao, B.L., Guo, Q. and Xin, W.J. (2001) Free radical scavenging by green tea polyphenols. *Method Enzymol.* **335**, 217–231.

Zhao, G., Vaszar, L.T., Qiu, D., Shi, L. and Kao, P.N. (2000) Anti-inflammatory effects of triptolide in human bronchial epithelial cells. *Am. J. Physiol. Lung. C.* **279**, 958–966.

Zhong, Z., Qu, Z., Wang, N., Wang, J., Xie, Z., Zhang, F., Zhang, W. and Lu, Z. (2005) Protective effects of Panax notoginseng saponins against pathological lesion of cholinergic neuron in rat model with Alzheimer' s disease. *Zhong Yao Cai* **28**, 119–122.

Zhou, H.F., Liu, X.Y., Niu, D.B., Li, F.Q., He, Q.H. and Wang, X.M. (2005) Triptolide protects dopaminergic neurons from inflammationmediated damage induced by lipopolysaccharide intranigral injection. *Neurobiol. Dis.* **18**, 441–449.

Zhou, Y. and Xu, R. (1992) Antioxidative effect of Chinese drugs. *Zhongguo Zhong Yao Za Zhi* **17**,368–369.

Zhu, W.W., Liu, Z.L., Xu, H.W., Chu, W.Z., Ye, Q.Y., Xie, A.M., Chen, L. and Li, J.R. (2005) Effect of the oil from *ganoderma lucidum* spores on pathological changes in the substantia nigra and behaviors of MPTP-treated mice. *Di Yi Jun Yi Da Xue Xue Bao* **25**, 667–671.

Chapter 8

Insomnia and Aging

Yun-Kwok Wing and Siu-Ping Lam

Abstract

Sleep is an essential and universal process for human being. There are progressive changes in sleep architecture, quality and quantity with advancing age. In addition, elderly has increased number of co-morbid illnesses that could further exacerbate their sleep changes. Insomnia is one of the commonest sleep problems in elderly, with a prevalence rate ranged from 23% to 38%. It is more common among female and highly co-morbid with physical and mental illnesses. Various factors contribute to insomnia including genetic, stress, physical and mental conditions, cognitive and neurobiological hyperarousal response. Hence, an integrated approach focusing on both insomnia and co-morbid illnesses is important when managing insomnia in elderly. In western medicine, in addition to pharmacological treatment there is concrete evidence that non-pharmacological approach such as sleep hygiene and cognitive behavioral therapy has promising results in the integrated treatment of insomnia. Traditional Chinese Medicine (TCM) and other alternative medicines such as acupuncture are other widely adopted treatment modalities. There has been a longstanding historical record of usage of various TCM formulae in treating insomnia or similar condition. Emerging evidence from modern practices suggested that some TCM formulae are effective in combating insomniac symptoms, such as the popular formula, Suan Zao Ren Tong. However, further clinical studies with modern scientific principles are needed in the study of TCM in the treatment of insomnia with respect to their safety and efficacy.

Keywords: Insomnia; Elderly; Traditional Chinese Medicine.

8.1 Introduction

Sleep is an essential biological process among all species, albeit the function of sleep has not yet been fully elucidated. It is a state characterized by a series of active dynamic physiological changes in neurological, cardiovascular, respiratory and endocrine systems. With advancing age, there are progressive changes in sleep architecture, quality and quantity of sleep. Various pathologies of sleep conditions could arise or exacerbate with aging. This chapter provides an overview of the sleep physiology, epidemiology, aetiology and management of insomnia in elderly population, particularly with reference to the management perspectives from both the Western and Traditional Chinese Medicine (TCM) aspects.

8.2 Sleep Physiology with Advancing Age

Sleep consists of alternate cycles of non rapid-eye-movement (NREM) sleep and rapid-eye-movement (REM) sleep as defined by electroencephalography (EEG), electro-oculography (EOG) and electromyography (EMG). NREM sleep is further classified into light sleep (stage 1 and stage 2) and slow wave sleep (SWS, stage 3). In human adult, each sleep cycle lasts for about 60–90 minutes with typically 4–6 cycles of NREM-REM sleep per night. Throughout the night, there is a progressive increase in REM sleep duration in each cycle (Fig. 8.1(a): normal hypnogram). Multiple neurotransmitters and hormones are responsible for the control of sleep-wake transition. The complex sleep cycles and propensity to sleep are tightly controlled by both homeostatic and circadian factors. Circadian rhythm is determined by the internal biological clock (suprachiasmatic nucleus of hypothalamus) and external cues especially light. This two-process model (circadian and homeostatsis) is postulated to be the fundamental regulation of our sleep process (Borbely, 1982).

The sleep architecture progressively changes across age with decrease in sleep duration, lesser SWS, more light sleep and increased sleep fragmentation (Fig. 8.1(b): hypnogram of an elderly). In parallel with the decrease in structured daytime activities, elderly people commonly have earlier bed-time and wake-up time. The understanding of these physiological changes in elderly sleep is important for both diagnostic and

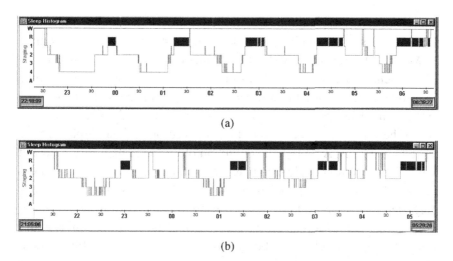

(a)

(b)

Fig. 8.1. (a) Hypnogram of an adult showing sleep cycles of NREM (Stages 1–4) and REM (R) sleep, with progressive increase in duration REM sleep and shortening of slow wave sleep (Stages 3 and 4). (b) Hypnogram of an elderly: advanced sleep phase increased sleep latency, fragmentation of sleep and decreased slow wave sleep (Stages 3 and 4, now renamed as stage 3 under the new scoring criteria; Iber *et al.*, 2007) (W: wake).

management aspects, making the emphasis of sleep hygiene as an important component in the management of elderly insomnia.

8.3 Insomnia in the Elderly: Clinical Epidemiology

In parallel with the physiological changes in sleep architecture, sleep disturbances with difficulties in falling and maintaining sleep are common among elderly. A local epidemiological survey of elderly population in Hong Kong Chinese (age >70) found out that 75% of subjects reported occasional or persistent sleep disturbances (Chiu *et al.*, 1999). However, not all elderly perceived these changes as insomniac complaints.

Insomnia is defined as a subjective complaint about sleep continuity, duration, or quality that results in daytime consequences. It could be classified as different subtypes- difficulty in initiating sleep, difficulty in maintaining sleep, waking up too early, or non-restorative sleep. Currently, there are a few international diagnostic criteria of insomnia, such as the

International Classification of Sleep Disorder (ICSD-II) (American Academy of sleep medicine, 2005) and Diagnostic and Statistical Manual of Mental Disorders (DSM-IV-TR) (American Psychiatric Association, 1994). Generally, a diagnosis of insomnia is defined as having any subtype of insomnia of at least three nights per week with consequent daytime impairment. The insomnia diagnosis may be further classified as according to the duration of illness and the presence of associated physical or mental conditions. Although the definition of insomnia may vary, research works from different clinical and general population have been carried out extensively. In elderly populations, worldwide epidemiological surveys suggested that the prevalence rate of insomnia ranged from 23% to 38% (Chiu *et al.*, 1999; Morgan *et al.*, 1988; Livingston *et al.*; Brabbins *et al.*, 1999; Henderson *et al.*, 1995; Foley *et al.*, 1995; Blazer *et al.*, 1995). As in adult populations, insomnia is more common among elderly females than males. (Zhang and Wing, 2006). With advancing age, there seems to have a higher prevalence of insomnia among elderly. Is insomnia related to an aging process? Recent evidence suggested that the prevalence of primary insomnia is actually relatively low in healthy older adults. (Foley *et al.*, 1999; 2004). Instead of age, comorbidities of physical and mental illnesses are the important factors associated with symptomatic insomnia (Chiu *et al.*, 1999). Regarding the course of insomnia, longitudinal studies suggested that insomnia often runs a persistent and chronic course, especially for those with more severe insomniac symptoms (Ganguli *et al.*, 1996; Morin *et al.*, 2009; Fong and Wing, 2007).

8.4 Insomnia: Comorbidities, Differential Diagnosis and Consequences

Insomnia is commonly described as a symptom secondary to other physical or mental problems. However, the limited understanding of the pathophysiological pathways of insomnia precludes the conclusions about the causality between insomniac symptoms and the medical or mental illnesses. Hence, recent expert consensus advocated the term of "co-morbid insomnia" instead of "secondary insomnia" (NIH, 2005).

It has long been recognized that insomnia is one of the most common presentations of mental illnesses such as depression and anxiety. The co-occurrence of insomnia and mental disorders were found to be up to 40% in general population (Ford and Kamerow, 1989; Roth *et al.*, 2006) and nearly 80% of sufferers of active depression complained of insomnia (Ohayon *et al.*, 2000). Apart from being a concurrent symptom, longitudinal follow-up studies suggested that insomnia is a predictor of future psychiatric illnesses, such as depression, anxiety disorders and alcohol dependence (Fong and Wing, 2007; Ford and Kamerow, 1989; Breslau *et al.*, 1996; Taylor *et al.*, 2005). These findings had been replicated in elderly populations (Roberts *et al.*, 2000; Mallon *et al.*, 2000). Insomnia has also been reported to be prevailing among various medical conditions. The prevalence of insomnia ranged from 30% to 70% in clinical populations with chronic heart failure, malignancy and chronic pain conditions (Katz and McHorney, 1998; Brostrom and Johansson, 2005; Savard and Morin, 2001; Stiefel and Stagno, 2004). The direct impact of physical symptoms, concurrent emotional distress and adverse effect of treatment may jointly contribute to insomnia.

Apart from psychiatric and medical disorders, insomnia could also be a disguise or associated condition of other sleep disorders, namely sleep apnea, circadian rhythm disorder and narcolepsy. Sleep apnea is characterized by recurrent episodes of upper airway obstruction with oxygen desaturation. Commonly presented with snoring and daytime sleepiness, insomnia could also be a common presentation, especially in female population (Shepertycky *et al.*, 2005). Thus, comorbid insomnia and sleep apnea poses treatment difficulties and compliance problem to continuous positive airway pressure (CPAP) treatment. Circadian rhythm embraces a variety of sleep disorders including advance/delay sleep phase syndrome, and common conditions such as jet lag and shift work. While some disorders (e.g. jet lag) could be transient, others could be a long-standing problem and mistaken as insomniac complaints.

The negative consequences of insomnia could not be neglected. Fatigue and poor concentration are common daytime complaints among chronic insomniacs (Stepanski *et al.*, 1988). In elderly populations, insomnia was found to be associated with increased risk of fall (Stone *et al.*, 2008). Studies have reported that poor sleepers were more likely to have motor-vehicle or other accidents compared to the good sleepers (NIH, 2005; Daley *et al.*, 2009). Work absenteeism and impaired work performance have also been found to be more common among people with insomnia (Daley *et al.*, 2009; Godet-Cayre *et al.*, 2006; Ozminkowski *et al.*, 2007). The health care utilization, direct and indirect costs of insomnia was substantial but the estimation was further complicated by its tight associations with various physical and mental problems.

8.5 Etiology of Insomnia

The development of insomnia could be conceptualized as a condition in which predisposing factors, precipitating events and perpetuating issues play interactive roles in the onset and maintenance of the insomniac symptoms. Being a disease with complex phenotypes, insomnia is likely to be regulated by multiple genes and environmental interactions. Genetic predisposition of insomnia has been suggested by the familial aggregation (Zhang *et al.*, 2009; Drake *et al.*, 2008) and high concordance rates in monozygotic twin pairs (Watson *et al.*, 2006). Acute stresses such as life events, changes in physical state, environmental or occupational aspects precipitate the insomniac symptoms. The onset and persistence of insomnia is further modulated and perpetuated by cognitive and neurobiological hyperarousal responses. (Riemann *et al.*, 2010). Cognitively, insomniac subjects tend to ruminate, become more attentive to the sleep complaints and daytime consequences of insomnia. Together with the maladaptive behaviors and poor sleep hygiene (like spending too much time lying awake at bed with ruminations and worryings), these may contribute to the learned conditioning associations between the bed and wakefulness, which further contribute to persistent insomniac symptoms. There are also evidences of somatic and autonomic hyperarousal among insomniacs, such as increased cortical activities, increased heart rate variability and neuro-hormonal disturbances, which play important mediating roles in both acute and chronic insomnia.

8.6 Management of Insomnia in Elderly

8.6.1 *Assessment of insomnia*

As insomnia is such a complex condition with tight associations of physical and mental comorbidities, early recognition, detailed assessment and treatment of both sleep and comorbid conditions by an integrated approach should be adopted. A comprehensive assessment should include a thorough medical, psychiatric, sleep histories and review on medication usage, including alcohol and caffeine intake. Details about the insomniac complaint, pattern, severity, and potential precipitating and perpetuating factors should be obtained. Apart from the nighttime symptoms, daytime symptoms including fatigue, attention problems and functional impairment are equally important in the clinical assessment.

To supplement the assessment, tools such as sleep logs or sleep diaries could be used for collection of daily information on sleep habits and clarification of the insomniac complaint. A comprehensive history, however, is mandatory and irreplaceable in the diagnosis and planning of therapeutic options for insomnia. Laboratory tests such as overnight polysomnography is rarely indicated for the assessment of insomnia, and it is usually reserved for complex cases, such as treatment resistant insomnia or suspicion of other comorbid sleep disorders, such as sleep apnea syndrome.

8.6.2 *Treatment — approach from western medicine perspectives*

In western medicine, insomnia is regarded as a complex condition contributed by both psycho-physiological and behavioral factors, hence, a variety of treatment modalities have been suggested, including pharmacological treatment and non-pharmacological approaches, such as general measures of sleep hygiene, relaxation, and cognitive behavioral therapy.

8.6.2.1 *Non-pharmacological management of insomnia*

Non-pharmacological intervention plays a key role in the management of chronic insomnia. Accumulating evidences suggested that psychological and behavioral treatment produced robust and sustained improvements in sleep continuity in both adult and elderly populations (Morin *et al.*, 2006; 2009; Riemann, 2009). There are various components of psychological and behavioral treatments, including sleep hygiene, general behavior technique of relaxation and cognitive behavioral therapy.

Sleep hygiene refers to issues about modifying lifestyle and sleep environment for better sleep. It is not only applicable to poor sleepers but also to everyone as healthy habits. An important but commonly neglected component of sleep hygiene is to build up a regular sleep-wake schedule. Although it seems to be a simple principle, most insomniac patients fail to master this basic rule and they frequently have chaotic or irregular sleep-wake schedule. Modifications in lifestyle include regular exercise, limiting the excessive consumption of caffeine, nicotine and alcohol. A comfortable bedroom environment is another important aspect for a good sleep, such as optimal temperature, lighting control, suitable pillows and mattress. Relaxation is a general tip for better sleep. It could range from practical advice of winding down and setting up pre-sleep routines to relaxation exercise, aiming at smoothing and de-arousal.

Apart from general sleep hygiene advice, cognitive behavioral therapy (CBT) is now one of the mainstay treatments for insomnia. CBT is a psychotherapeutic method based on the theory that one's own distorted thoughts and beliefs contribute to emotional and behavioral problems. CBT works by helping one to realize and change his/her unhealthy belief and attitude, to re-interpret the events in a more rational and realistic way. Dysfunctional beliefs and attitudes about sleep have been well documented among patients with insomnia (Morin *et al.*, 1993) and some examples were listed in Table 8.1. The common pitfalls among insomniacs

Table 8.1. Common dysfunctional beliefs about insomnia (Adapted from The Dysfunctional Beliefs and Attitudes about Sleep Scale DBAS by Morin (1994))

---

1. Rumination of the consequences of insomnia
   I cannot function at all after a poor night's sleep!
2. Unrealistic expectation about sleep
   I must have 8 hours of sleep every night!
3. Concerns about control over sleep
   I am losing control over my abilities to fall asleep!
   My sleep problem is getting so bad that nothing can help!
4. Misconceptions about sleep-promoting practices
   I should try harder if I can't fall asleep right away!

Table 8.2. Stimulus control therapy for insomnia.

1. Avoid using the bed for activities other than sleep and sex
2. Go to bed only when you are sleepy
3. Get out of your bed if you can't fall asleep
4. Keep a regular sleep-wake schedule
5. Avoid napping in the daytime

are having unrealistic and faulty attributions about sleep and consequences of insomnia. These misconceptions further contribute to emotional distress and maladaptive habits, and hence perpetuate the insomniac problems. The cognitive therapy on insomnia helps the insomniac to build up a more rational and realistic perspectives, to strengthen their sense of control and to develop healthy coping skills. In parallel with working on cognitive aspects, changes on behavior should also be emphasized in order to maximize treatment effects. Stimulus control and sleep restriction are the two specific behavioral management for insomnia. (Table 8.2) To have a good night sleep, an appropriate and discriminative stimuli of the bedroom environment is important. Insomnia result from failure to establish such stimuli or presence of inappropriate stimuli that are incompatible to sleep. Poor stimulus control such as habits of eating or working at bedroom, will gradually create a learned association between bed and wakefulness. Stimulus control therapy emphasize the restoration of appropriate stimuli and deconditioning the wakeful stimuli with beds. Sleep restriction is another important behavioral modification among insomniac patients. Instead of staying awake in bed for long hours as most insomniacs do, sleep restriction emphasize the importance of having a higher efficiency of sleep by reducing one's bedtime hours close to the perceived subjective sleep time. When a sleep pattern of higher sleep efficiency established, a gradual lengthening of bedtime could be introduced.

8.6.2.2 *Pharmacological treatment*

Although there is increasing emphasis on cognitive behavioral management of insomnia, pharmacological treatment remains on the top of the intervention list among many insomniac subjects (Walsh and Schweitzer,

1999). Commonly available prescription drugs from western medicine include benzodiazepine, non-benzodiazepine hypnotics, antidepressants, and anti-histamine drugs. An ideal hypnotic should be short-acting, with good tolerability and minimal drug dependence profile. Many of the currently available sedative-hypnotics fall short of these criteria, while some off-label prescription drugs, such as antidepressants and anti-histamine drugs, lack concrete evidence in supporting their safety and effectiveness in the management of insomnia. The characteristics and common side effects are listed in Table 8.3.

8.6.3 *Role of Traditional Chinese Medicine (TCM) in the management of insomnia*

The clinical significance of insomnia was first described in the earliest TCM records nearly two thousand years ago, such as *Ling Shu* (circa 200AD)

Table 8.3. Common types of western medication for insomnia.

Drugs	Examples	Proposed mechanism	Duration of action	Side effects
Benzodiazepine	Bromazepam Lorazepam Diazepam	Gamma-aminobutyric acid system (GABA)	Ultra-short to long acting	Somnolence, hangover, amnesia, abuse and dependence
Non-Benzodiazepine	Zolpidem Zopiclone	Gamma-aminobutyric acid system (GABA)	Ultra-short to short acting	Drowsiness, somnolence
Antidepressants (low dose)	Trazodone Doxepin	Adrenergic and histaminergic	Long-acting	Somnolence, headache, cardiac events
Antihistamines	Chloramphenamine Promethazine Diphenhydramine	Histaminergic and cholinergic	Long-acting	Somnolence, dry mouth, urinary retention

and Golden Chest (circa 300AD) (Wing, 2001; Quan *et al.*, 2001; Zhang, 1967; Wang, 1936). According to the TCM concept, normal body functioning involves regulation of *yin* and *yang*, as well as the interactions of five basic elements and the vital organs as according to *Wu Hsing* theory (Wing, 2001). The disturbances of homeostasis of these balances would give rise to illnesses. Upon appropriate treatment, the balance between *yin* and *yang* could be restored and the flow of *qi*, blood and body fluids could be normalized. For example, according to the standard TCM approach, insomnia is caused mainly by four types of disturbances: deficiency of the heart and spleen-*qi*, disharmony between the heart and kidney, upward disturbance of the liver fire, and finally dysfunctions of the stomach (Wing, 2001). These factors may jointly contribute to insomnia. This interesting theoretical TCM perspective on insomnia certainly needs further empirical evaluation and comparison with the western medicinal perspective. However, at this moment, there is very limited direct comparison of both western medicinal and TCM approach in the diagnosis of insomnia.

The use of alternative medicine for insomnia is common and under-investigated. A national poll in United States in 2005 reported that about 9% of the respondents consumed over-the-counter (OTC) medicine for their sleep problems (National Sleep Foundation, 2005). In Hong Kong, over 40% of the insomniac subjects reported the use of herbs for treatment of their illnesses (Fong, unpublished data). In this regard, herbal medicine of both western and TCM origins are the most common ingredients of OTC medications in Hong Kong (Wing, 2001; Chung and Lee, 2002). Nonetheless, a major difference between western herbal and TCM products is that the western herb is usually in isolated form while a typical TCM treatment is based on a composite formula. The rationale for combining various herbal products in the TCM treatment is based on the belief that different herbs may serve as various functions in the formula such as 'Master', 'Soldier' and 'Adviser' (Wing, 2001; Chan, 1995). Tables 8.4 and 8.5 shows the common TCM herbs, ingredients and formulae in Hong Kong.

In fact, some of these herbs were shown to have sedative effects in both animal and human studies (Wing, 2001; Wang et al., 2007). Although the exact mechanism is still obscure, some TCM products were thought to exert their sedative effects via similar mechanisms as in western sedative-hypnotics, such as acting on the gamma aminobutyric acid

Table 8.4. Common TCM herbs/ingredients for treatment of insomnia in Hong Kong (Adapted with permission from the Hong Kong Medical Journal, Wing et al., 2001. Copyright year 2001, Hong Kong Academy of Medicine).

Bontanical Product	Name	Traditional Chinese medicine rationale for use/indication	主治
Fruit 果實種子類	Suanzaoren (Semen Ziziphi Spinosae) 酸棗仁	To nourish the heart, benefit the liver and tranquilize the mind. For vexation, insomnia, severe palpitation, frightening and amnesia	養心益肝、寧心安神 治心煩失眠、驚悸征忡、健忘
	Dazao (Fructus Jujubae) 大棗	To revitalize the spleen and stomach. For blood-deficiency with insomnia	補益脾胃 養血安神：治血虛失眠
	Longyanrou (Arillus Longan) 眼肉	To revitalize the heart and spleen, nourish blood and calm the mind. For palpitation, insomnia, amnesia and dizziness	補益心脾、養血安神 治氣血虛所致驚悸征忡、失眠、健忘、眩暈
	Baiziren (Platycladi Semen) 柏子仁	To nourish the heart and tranquilize the mind. For frightening, severe palpitation, dreaminess amnesia and night sweating	養心安神 治心血不足之驚悸、征忡、失眠多夢、健忘、虛汗
	Wuweizi (Schisandrae Fructus) 五味子	To benefit vital energy and invigorate kidney, nourish the heart and calm the mind. For palpitation, insomnia and frequent dreams	益氣生津、斂肺氣止咳喘補腎固澀 養心安神 治心虛之悸、失眠、多夢

(Continued)

Table 8.4. (*Continued*)

Bontanical Product	Name	Traditional Chinese medicine rationale for use/indication	主治
	Fuxiaomai (*Tritici Fructus Levis*) 浮小麥	Nourish the heart and tranquilize the mind For palpitation, insomnia and dreaminess	養心安神 治心血不足之婦人,臟躁、神志恍 惚、失眠、多夢等
Root and Rhizome 根及根莖類	*Banzia* (*Pinelliae Rhizoma*) 半夏	To deprive dampness and disperse stagnation To eliminate toxic material, disperse lumps and relieve carbuncle	燥濕化痰 消痞散結;外敷攻毒散結消癰
	Danshen (*Salviae Miltiorrhizae Radix*) 丹參	To promote blood circulation to remove blood stasis, clear away heat, relieve vexation, nourish blood and tranquilize the mind For restlessness, frightening and insomnia	活血袪瘀、清熱除煩、養血安神 治心熱或心血不足之心神不安、驚 悸、失眠
	Chaihu (*Bupleuri Radix*) 柴胡	To disperse the stagnated liver energy and to increase yang-energy	解表洩熱、清透少陽邪熱、疏肝解 鬱、升舉陽氣
	Danggui (*Radix Angelicae Sinensis*) 當歸	To enrich blood and promote blood circulation	補血

(*Continued*)

Table 8.4. (*Continued*)

Bontanical Product	Name	Traditional Chinese medicine rationale for use/indication	主治
	Baizhu (*Atractylodis Macrocephalae Rhizoma*) 白朮	To invigorate the spleen and benefit vital energy	補脾益氣
Cortex皮類	*Hehuanpi* (*Albizziae Cortex*) 合歡皮	To tranquilize the mind and disperse the depressed vital energy For emotional upset, depression, insomnia, and amnesia	安神解鬱 治七情所致精神忿怒憂鬱、虛煩不眠、健忘等
Rattan藤 木類	*Shouwuteng* (*Polygoni Caulis*) 首烏藤 / 夜交藤	To nourish the heart and tranquilize the mind For vexation, insomnia, dreaminess and insanity	養心安神 治陰虛血少的虛煩、失眠、多夢
Fungus菌 藻類	*Lingzhi* (*Ganoderma*) 靈芝	To tranquilize the mind, enrich vital energy and blood For insomnia, dreams	養心安神，補益血氣 用於心氣虛或心血虛之失眠、多夢
	Fuling (*Poria*) 茯苓	To promote diuresis To invigorate the spleen To tranquilize the mind	利水滲濕，健脾補中 養心安神：心脾兩虛或痰飲所致心悸、失眠

Table 8.5. Common TCM formulae for insomnia treatment in Hong Kong. (Adapted with permission from the Hong Kong Medical Journal 2001, Wing, *et al.*, 2001. Copyright year 2001, Hong Kong Academy of Medicine).

Name	Ingredients	藥物組成
Liquorice, Wheat	*Radix Glycyrrhizae*	甘草
and Jujuba Soup	*Triticum Aestivum*	小麥
甘麥大棗湯	*Fructus Ziziphus Jujuba*	大棗
Suan Zao Ren Tang	*Semen Zizyphi Spinosae*	酸棗仁
酸棗仁湯	*Sclerotium Poriae Cocos*	茯苓
	Radix Ligustici Wallichii	川芎
	Rhizoma Anemarrhenea Aspheloidis	知母
	Radix Glycyrrhizae	甘草
Xiao Yao Wan	*Radix Bupleuri*	柴胡
逍遙丸	*Radix Angelica Sinensis*	當歸
	Radix Albus Paeoniae Lactiflorae	白芍
	Rhizoma Atractylodis Macrocephalae	白朮
	Sclerotium Poriae Cocos	茯苓
	Radx Glycyrrhizae	甘草
	Herba Menthae haplocalycis	薄荷
	Uncooked *Rhizoma Zingiberis*	生乾薑

(GABA) and serotonin (5-HT) system (Wing, 2001; Wang et al., 2007). Among these TCM formulae, the best known one is the Suanzaoren Tang, which contains Semen ziziphi spinosae, Sclerotium poriae cocos, Radix ligustici wallichii, Rhizoma anemarrhenea aspheloidis, and mix-fried Radix glycyrrhizae. It has undergone several clinical trials including large clinical case series and double-blind case controlled studies. There are some encouraging results that Suanzaoren Tang might be effective in treating insomnia (Yu, 1965; Zhang et al., 2000). However, more well-established clinical trials and pharmacological studies would be needed to ascertain the definitive role of TCM in the management of insomnia.

8.6.4 *Acupuncture for insomnia*

Acupuncture is another common treatment modality for insomnia that was originated in China over 2000 years ago (Wu, 1996). The traditional method of acupuncture is done by inserting fine needles over the meridian points which govern different parts of body. With modernization, various forms of acupuncture have been developed, such as electro-acupuncture, laser acupuncture and auricular therapy. Although acupuncture has been a common complementary treatment for both Chinese and Western populations for a variety of illnesses, its efficacy on management of insomnia has not been finally established. A recent review article concluded that despite the increasing published data on acupuncture for insomnia, there was still no firm conclusion about its efficacy, as the number of randomized controlled studies was limited with heterogeneous recruitment and study designs (Yeung *et al.*, 2009; Cheuk, 2007).

8.6.5 *Current limitations on the use of TCM for insomnia*

Although TCM is a popular treatment option of insomnia in a number of countries, its risk benefit ratio has not been clearly demarcated. Cautions are needed in some formulae e.g. Cinnabaris in *Zhu Sha An Shen Wan*, which contains heavy metal like mercury and carries risk of cumulative toxicity on prolonged usage (Wing, 2001; Wei *et al.*, 1999). To establish the effectiveness of a treatment, there has been an emphasis of evidence-based data in modern western medical practice. The commonly employed golden standard in judging the clinical efficacy of a treatment is based on well conducted randomized clinical trials, especially with placebo-control design. In this regard, most TCM products in the treatment of insomnia have been largely based on clinical experiences and open case series, while randomized placebo-controlled studies were very limited (Wing, 2001). In order to establish the efficacy and safety of TCM for insomnia, collaborations between the western science and the Oriental knowledge are important, including the use of evidence based medicine in TCM by well-designed randomized control studies.

8.7 Conclusion

Insomnia is a prevalent condition among elderly. Instead of a simple aging process, it is commonly associated with physical and mental disorders. The negative consequences and longitudinal course of chronicity could not be underestimated. There are a variety of treatment options, ranging from sleep hygiene, psychological and behavioral therapy, drug therapy from both Western and Chinese medicine. An integrated approach of both pharmacological and non-pharmacological measures is suggested in combating insomnia. For western medications, short term clinical efficacy has been established in some of the commonly used sedatives but long term efficacy and safety among elderly populations is still lacking. Further works are needed to establish the efficacy and safety of TCM therapy including use of various herbal formulae and acupuncture in the elderly as well as the combination of both western and TCM management of insomnia.

References

American Academy of Sleep Medicine. (2005) *The International Classification of Sleep Disorders, Diagnostic and Coding Manual*, 2nd edn. American Academy of Sleep Medicine: Westchester, Illinois.

American Psychiatric Association. (1994) *Diagnostic and Statistical Manual of Mental Disorder*, 4th edn. American Psychiatric Association, Washington, DC.

Blazer, D.G., Hays, J.C. and Foley, D.J. (1995) Sleep complaints in older adults: A racial comparison. *J. Gerontol. A-Biol.* **50A**, M280–M284.

Borbely, A.A. (1982) A two-process model of sleep regulation. *Hum. Neurobiol.* **1**, 195–204.

Brabbins, C.J., Dewey, M.E., Copeland, J.R.M., *et al.* (1999) Insomnia in the elderly: Prevalence, gender differences and relationships with morbidity and mortality. *Int. J. Geriat. Psych.* **8**, 473–480.

Breslau, N., Roth, T., Rosenthal, L. and Andreski, P. (1996) Sleep disturbance and psychiatric disorders: A longitudinal epidemiological study of young adults. *Biol. Psychiat.* **39**, 411–418.

Brostrom, A. and Johansson, P. (2005) Sleep disturbances in patients with chronic heart failure and their holistic consequence — what different care actions can be implemented. *Eur. J. Cardiovasc. Nur.* **4**(3), 183–197.

Chan, K. Progress in traditional Chinese medicine. (1995) Trends *Pharmacol. Sci.* **16**, 182–187.

Cheuk, D.K.L., Yeung, J., Chung, K.F. and Wong, V. (2007) Acupuncture for insomnia. *Cochrane Database Syst. Rev.* **18**(3), CD005472.

Chiu, H.F., Leung, T., Lam, L.C., *et al.* (1999) Sleep problems in Chinese elderly in Hong Kong. *Sleep* **22**(6), 717–726.

Chung, K.F. and Lee, C.K.Y. (2002) Over-the-counter sleeping pills: A survey of use in Hong Kong and a review of their constituents. *Gen. Hosp. Psychiat.* **24**, 430–435.

Daley, M., Morin, C.M., LeBlanc, M., Gregoire, J.P., Savard, J. and Baillargeon, L. (2009) Insomnia and its relationship to health-care utilization, work absenteeism, productivity and accidents. *Sleep Med.* **10**, 427–438.

Drake, C.L., Scofield, H. and Roth, T. (2008) Vulnerability to insomnia: the role of familial aggregation. *Sleep Med.* **9**, 297–302.

Foley, D., Ancoli-Israel, S., Britz, P. and Walsh, J. (2004) Sleep disturbances and chronic disease in older adults: Results of the 2003 National Sleep Foundation Sleep in America Survey. *J. Psychosom. Res.* **56**(5), 497–502.

Foley, D.J., Monjan, A., Simonsick, E.M., Wallace, R.B. and Blazer, D.G. (1999) Incidence and remission of insomnia among elderly adults: An epidemiologic study of 6,800 persons over three years. *Sleep* **22**(Suppl. 2), S366–S372.

Foley, D.J., Monjan, A.A., Brown, S.L., *et al.* (1995) Sleep complaints among elderly persons: An epidemiologic study of three communities. *Sleep* **18**, 425–432.

Fong, S.Y.Y. and Wing, Y.K. (2007) Longitudinal follow up of a primary insomnia patients in a psychiatric clinic. *Aust. NZ J. Psychiat.* **41**, 611–617.

Ford, D. E. and Kamerow, D.B. (1989) Epidemiologic study of sleep disturbances and psychiatric disorders. An opportunity for prevention? *J. Am. Med. Assoc.* **262**, 1479–1484.

Ganguli, M., Reynolds, C.F. and Gilby, J.E. (1996) Prevalence and persistence of sleep complaints in a rural older community sample: The MoVIES project. *J. Am. Geriatr. Soc.* **44**(7), 778–784.

Godet-Cayre, V., Pelletier-Fleury, N., Le Vaillant, M., *et al.* (2006) Insomnia and absenteeism at work. Who pays the cost? *Sleep* **29**, 179–184.

Henderson, S., Jorm, A.F., Scott, L.T., *et al.* (1995) Insomnia in the elderly: Its prevalence and correlates in the general population. *Med. J. Aust.* **162**, 22–24.

Iber, C., Ancoli-Israel, S., Chesson, A., *et al.* (2007) *The AASM Manual for the Scoring of Sleep and Associated Events: Rules, Terminology and Technical Specifications*, 1st edn. American Academy of Sleep Medicine, Westchester, Illinois.

Katz, D.A. and McHorney, C.A. (1998) Clinical correlates of insomnia in patients with chronic illness. *Arch. Int. Med.* **158**, 1099–1107.

Livingston, G., Hawkins, A., Graham, N., *et al.* (1990) The Gospel Oak study: Prevalence rate of dementia, depression and activity limitation among elderly residents in Inner London. *Psychol. Med.* **20**, 137–146.

Mallon, L., Broman, J.E. and Hetta, J. (2000) Relationship between insomnia, depression and mortality: 1 12-year follow-up of older adults in community. *Int. Psychogeriatr.* **12**, 295–306.

Morgan, K., Dallosso, H., Ebrahim, S., *et al.* (1988) Characteristics of subjective insomnia among the elderly living at home. *Age Ageing* **17**, 1–7.

Morin, C.M. (1994) Dysfunctional beliefs and attitudes about sleep: preliminary scale development and description. *Behav. Ther.* **17**, 163–164.

Morin, C.M., Belanger, L., LeBlanc, M., Ivers, H., Savard, J., Espie, C.A., Merette, C., Baillargeon, L. and Gregoire J.P. (2009) The natural history of insomnia. *Arch. Int. Med.* **169**(5), 447–453.

Morin, C.M., Bootzin, R.R., Buysse, D.J., Edinger, J.D., Espie, C.A. and Lichstein K.L. (2006) Psychological and behavioral treatment of insomnia: an update of the recent evidence. 1998–2004. *Sleep* **29**, 1398–1414.

Morin, C.M., Stone, J., Trinkle, D., Mercer, J. and Remsberg, S. (1993) Dysfunctional beliefs and attitudes about sleep among older adults with and without insomnia complaints. *Psychol. Aging* **8**, 463–467.

Morin, C.M., Vallieres, A., Guay, B., Ivers, H., Savard, J., Merette, C., Bastien, C. and Baillargeon, L. (2005) Cognitive behavioral therapy, singly and combined with medication, for persistent insomnia. A randomized controlled trial. *J. Am. Med. Assoc.* **301**, 2005–2015.

National Institutes of Health (2005) NIH State-of-the-Science Conference Statement on manifestations and management of chronic insomnia in adults. *NIH Consens. State. Sci. Statements* **22**(2), 1–30.

National Sleep Foundation. (2005) Sleep in America poll. http://www.sleepfoundation. org.

Ohayon, M.M., Shapiro, C.M. and Kennedy, S.H. (2000) Differentiating DSM-IV anxiety and depressive disorders in the general population: comorbidity and treatment consequences. *Can. J. Psychiat.* **45**, 166–172.

Ozminkowski, R.J., Shaohung, S.W. and Walsh, J.K. (2007) The direct and indirect costs of untreated insomnia in adults in the United States. *Sleep* **30**, 263–273.

Quan, S.J., Shi, T.X., Wang, S.G., *et al.* (2001) *Neurosis*, 1st edn. Tian Heng Wen Hua Publisher, Hong Kong.

Riemann, D. and Perlis, M.L. (2009) Treatment of chronic insomnia: A review of benzodiazepine receptor agonists and psychological and behavioral therapies. *Sleep Med. Rev.* **13**, 205–214.

Riemann, D., Spiegelhalder, K., Feige, B., Voderholzer, U., Berger, M., Perlis, M. and Nissen, C. (2010) The hyperarousal model of insomnia: A review of the concept and its evidence. *Sleep Med. Rev.* **14**, 19–31

Roberts, R.E., Shema, S.J., Kaplan, G.A. and Strawbridge, W.J. (2000) Sleep complaints and depression in an aging cohort: A prospective perspective. *Am. J. Psychiat.* **157**, 81–88.

Roth, T., Jaeger, S., Jin, R., Kalsekar, A., Stang, P.E. and Kessler, R.C. (2006) Sleep problems, comorbid mental disorders, and role functioning in National Comorbidity Survey Replication. *Bio. Psychiat.* **60**, 1364–1371.

Savard, J. and Morin, C.M. (2001) Insomnia in the context of cancer: A review of neglected problem. *J. Clin. Onco.* **19**, 895–908.

Shepertycky, M.R., Banno, K. and Kryger, M.H. (2005) Differences between men and women in the clinical presentation of patients diagnosed with obstructive sleep apnea syndrome. *Sleep* **28**, 309–314.

Stepanski, E., Zorick, F., Roehrs, T., *et al.* (1988) Daytime alertness in patients with chronic insomnia compared with asymptomatic control subjects. *Sleep* **11**, 54–60.

Stiefel, F. and Stagno, D. (2004) Management of insomnia in patients with chronic pain conditions. *CNS Drugs* **18**, 285–296.

Stone, L.K., Ensrud, K.E. and Ancoli-Israel, S. (2008) Sleep, insomnia and falls in elderly patient. *Sleep Med.* **9**, S18–S22

Taylor, D.J., Lichstein, K.L., Durrence, H.H., Reidel. B.W. and Bush, A.J. (2005) Epidemiology of insomnia, depression and anxiety. *Sleep* **28**, 1457–1464.

Walsh, J.K. and Schweitzer, P.K. (1999) Ten-year trends in the pharmacological treatment of insomnia. *Sleep* **22**, 371–375.

Wang, B. (1936) *Miraculous Pivot.* [In Chinese]. Zhonghua Shu Ju Shanghai.

Wang, Q., Wang, L.W. and Liu, X.M. (2007) Brief review about compatibility and their pharmacological effects of Chinese material medica as tranquilizer. [in Chinese] China *Journal of Chinese Materia Medica.* **32**(22), 2342–2346.

Watson, N.F., Goldberg, J., Arguelles, L. and Buchwald, D. (2006) Genetic and environmental influences on insomnia, daytime sleepiness, and obesity in twins. *Sleep* **29**, 645–649.

Wei, J.F., Shang, W.F. and Yang, S.L. (1999) The summary of pharmacology and toxicology of Cinnabaris [in Chinese]. *Chinese Traditional and Herbal Drugs* **30**, 954–945.

Wing, Y.K. (2001) Herbal treatment of insomnia. *Hong Kong Med. J.* **7**, 392–402.

Wu, J.N. (1996) A short history of acupuncture. *J. Altern. Complem. Med.* **2**, 19–21.

Yeung, W.F., Chung, K.F., Leung, Y.K., Zhang, S.P. and Lam, A.C.K. (2009) Traditional needle acupuncture treatment of insomnia: A systemic review of randomized controlled trials. *Sleep Med.* **10**, 694–704.

Yu, C.Z. (1965) The analysis of treatment of neurasthenia in different combinations of Suanzaoren Tang in 209 patients. *Shan Dong Yi Kan* **9**, 27.

Zhang, B. and Wing, Y.K. (2006) Sex differences in insomnia: A meta-analysis. *Sleep* **29**(1), 85–93.

Zhang, H., Cao, X.L., Sun, X.Q., *et al.* (2000) The treatment of insomnia of Anshen pill in 151 patients. *J. Tradit. Chin. Med.* **41**, 418–419.

Zhang, J., Li, A.M., Kong, A.P.S., Lai, K.Y.C., Tang, N.L.S. and Wing, Y.K. (2009) A community-based study of insomnia in Hong Kong Chinese children: prevalence, risk factors and familial aggregation. *Sleep Med.* **10**, 1040–1046.

Zhang, Z. (1967) *The Lecture Notes of the Synopsis of Prescriptions of the Golden Chamber* [in Chinese]. 1st edn. Yi Yao Wei Sheng Chu Ban She, Hong Kong.

Chapter 9

Study on the Mechanisms of Treating Stable Chronic Obstructive Pulmonary Disease with Bufeiyishen Granule

Jian-Sheng Li, Su-Yun Li, Ming-Hang Wang and Xue-Qing Yu

Abstract

Objective: To evaluate the therapeutic effect of *Bufeiyishen Granule* on chronic obstructive pulmonary disease (COPD) through clinical and experimental studies.

Methods: In the clinical study, 62 stable COPD patients were divided into treatment group and control group, treated for six months, and observed for changes of lung function and number of acute exacerbation. In the experimental study, 105 rats were randomly divided into seven groups (control group, stable model group, acute exacerbation model group, high-dose group, low-dose group, Flumucil group, and *Yupingfeng* group), and measured for routine blood test, artery blood gas, bronchoalveolar lavage fluid (BALF), lung function, pathological changes and matrix metalloproteinases (MMPs) at measurement points.

Results: In the clinical study, forced expiratory volume in one second, maximum mid-expiratory flow rate, peak expiratory volume and FEV1% were increased significantly ($p < 0.05$, $p < 0.01$), and the number of acute exacerbations was remarkably decreased ($p < 0.01$) in treatment group, but no obvious changes were found in control group. The experimental study showed higher leukocyte and neutrophil counts in the peripheral blood, bronchial BALF in the acute exacerbation model group, together with elevated levels of blood gas $PaCO_2$, MMP-9 and MMP-2, and worse lung function and blood gas PaO_2 as compared to the control and stable model groups; the low-dose group could improve the above changes.

Conclusion: *Bufeiyishen* Granule could improve the lung function in stable COPD patients and decrease the number of acute exacerbation. Animal models of stable COPD and acute exacerbation state were successfully created. *Bufeiyishen* Granule could also improve the changes of MMPs in COPD.

Keywords: Bufeiyishen Granule; Chronic Obstructive Pulmonary Disease (COPD); Animal Model; Clinical Research.

9.1 Introduction

Chronic obstructive pulmonary disease (COPD) is an incompletely reversible inflammatory disease of the respiratory tract. Its high morbidity, disability rate seriously impair the quality of life and activity of the patients, contributed to higher global economic burden of disease (Shreprek *et al.*, 2004). Airway inflammation and airway remodeling are the major pathological characteristics, repeated acute exacerbations in the course of the disease is the key factor leading to impairment of lung function, promotion of disease progression and airway remodeling. Cessation of smoking can ease the decrease in lung function. Long-term inhalation of β_2 agonists, corticosteroids, and anti-cholinergic drug can improve the reactivity of bronchus and relieve the impairment of the disease in severe patients, but these treatments are not able to be widely used in China due to the high cost. We have established the traditional Chinese medicine (TCM) treatment plan in the long-term treatment of COPD. We treated COPD patients in remission stage with *Bufeiyishen* Therapy (Tonifying the Lung and Reinforcing the Kidney) and observed its effects on lung function and acute exacerbation. There is a lack of suitable COPD animal model that can resemble clinical circumstances. A combination of cigarette smoke and bacteria intranasal injection were used to make COPD stable phase model; on the basis of model stability, a high dose of bacteria intranasal injection was performed to create the COPD acute exacerbation model, and the influences of *Bufeiyishen* Granule on metalloprotease in COPD rats was observed.

9.2 Part 1: Study on the Mechanisms of Treating Stable Chronic Obstructive Pulmonary Disease with *Bufeiyishen* Granule

9.2.1 *Method*

(1) **Study population:**

Stable phase of COPD outpatients.

(2) **Western medicine diagnosis and classification standard:**

Refer to the 2006 edition of *Chronic Obstructive Lung Disease Global Initiative (GOLD)* and the *Guidance of Diagnosis and Treatment of Chronic Obstructive Pulmonary Disease* issued by the Chinese Medical Association Respiratory Diseases Branch in January 2007. Severity of COPD should be evaluated according to the symptoms of patients, abnormality of lung function, existence of complications (such as respiratory failure, heart failure), in which the decrease of FEV_1 that reflect the airflow obstruction level is of great significance. There are four levels of COPD severity based on lung function (COPD team, 2007).

(3) **Traditional Chinese Medicine (TCM) syndrome classification of COPD:**

Syndrome of deficiency of lung-kidney *qi*: gasping, wheezing, coughing, shortness of breath, faint low voice, weak of waist and knees, tinnitus, dizzy, frequent micturition or dribble of urine or even enuresis, night excessive urinate, facial edema, pale tongue and white tongue coating, deep, thready pulse and weak pulse.

(4) **Inclusion criteria:**

Patients meeting the diagnostic criteria for COPD; syndrome of deficiency of lung-kidney *qi*; stable COPD patients with level I to level III severity, age ≥ 40 years, ≤ 80 years; not involved in any clinical trials for other drugs within one month; had underwent two weeks of washout period before selected; voluntarily participation in the treatment and signing of informed consent form.

(5) **Exclusion criteria:**

COPD acute exacerbation patients; COPD patients with level severity; pregnant and lactating women; patients with obnubilation, dementia, or other mental disorders; severe cardiac insufficiency; bronchial asthma, or bronchiectasis, or active tuberculosis; diffuse panbronchiolitis;

patients with pneumothorax, pleural effussion, pulmonary embolism; neuromuscular disease which affects respiratory movement functions; tumors; severe liver and kidney diseases; patients abed for long-term with any reasons; administered glucocorticoid within one month; congenital or acquired immunodeficiency; and allergy to the medicine used in this study.

(6) **Outcome measures:**

Number and severity of COPD acute exacerbation; pulmonary ventilation functions.

(7) **Treatment:**

Patients in treatment group took one dose of *Bufeiyishen* Granule (the manufacturer is up to the standard of Good Manufacturing Practice (GMP)). The herbal formula composition included *dangshen* (党参) 15 g, *huangqi* （黄芪）15 g, *shudi* (熟地) 9 g, *shanyurou* (山萸肉) 15 g, *wuweizi* (五味子) 9 g, *yinyanghuo* (淫羊藿) 15 g, *zhebeimu* (浙贝母) 9 g, *xiebai* (薤白) 9 g, *suzi* (苏子) 9 g, *chishao* (赤芍) 9 g, *dilong* (地) 9 g, *chenpi* (陈皮) 9 g, and *zhigancao* (炙甘草) 3 g), which was orally administrated in two times per day. Control group patients took placebos, with the same dose and administration as in treatment group; each course of medical treatment took three months, treatment effects were observed after two courses of treatments.

9.2.2 *Results*

From the Department of Respiratory Medicine, The Respiratory Disease Research Unit, First Affiliated Hospital of Henan University of Traditional Chinese Medicine more and Respiratory Disease Research Unit, Henan Provincial People's Hospital, 62 COPD patients who were in the remission stage were studied, excluding four patients with insufficient information, and another four who were not taking the medicine regularly. Based on the age, duration of the disease and severity, 62 patients who met the requirements of the study were randomly enrolled to treatment group and control group with 31 in each group. The treatment group had 23 males and eight females, age range from 57–76 (70.84 ± 6.78), with 18.38 ± 6.05 years duration of the disease; the control group had 24 males and seven females, age ranging from 58–77 (72.17 ± 7.17), with

Table 9.1. Influences of *Bufeiyishen* Granule in COPD lung ventilatory function $\bar{x} \pm s$).

	n		$FEV_{1.0}$ (L)	MMEF (L/s)	PEF (L/s)	$FEV_1\%$
Treatment group	31	before treatment	1.432 ± 0.400	0.778 ± 0.247	2.039 ± 0.843	50.619 ± 12.692
	31	after treatment	1.678 ± 0.499▲	0.888 ± 0.332▲	2.578 ± 1.531▲	61.729 ± 12.793▲
Control group	31	before treatment	1.437 ± 0.343	0.775 ± 0.226	1.991 ± 0.840	50.744 ± 12.757
	31	after treatment	1.367 ± 0.441	0.761 ± 0.258	2.010 ± 0.827	50.344 ± 14.192

Compare to control group before treatment: $p > 0.05$; compare to treatment group before treatment: $p < 0.05$, $p < 0.01$; compare to control group after treatment: ▲$p < 0.01$.

19.37 ± 6.24 years duration of the disease. There were nine patients in mild state of the illness, five in the treatment group and four in the control group; 42 patients were in moderate condition, with 21 in each group; six out of the 11 severe patients were in the treatment group, while the other five were in the control group.

9.2.2.1 *Changes in lung ventilatory function in the two groups (Table 9.1)*

After taking *Bufeiyishen* Granule for two months, patients in the treatment group had significant increases in forced expiratory volume in one second (FEV1.0), maximum mid-expiratory flow rate (MMEF) and peak expiratory volume (PEF), FEV1% ($p < 0.05$, $p < 0.01$). These parameters showed no obvious changes in control group; the spirometric parameters in treatment group showed better improvement than those in the control group ($p < 0.01$).

9.2.2.2 *Changes of number of acute exacerbation in the two groups*

After treatment, patients in treatment group had significant decreases in the number of COPD acute exacerbations ($p < 0.01$), patients in the control group showed no obvious change in the number of acute exacerbations.

	n		AECOPD number
Treatment group	31	before treatment	2.8 ± 1.2
	31	after treatment	0.6 ± 0.5▲
Control group	31	before treatment	2.7 ± 2.1
	31	after treatment	2.8 ± 2.5

Compare to control group before treatment: $p > 0.05$; compare to treatment group before treatment $p < 0.05$, $p < 0.01$; compare to control group after treatment: ▲$p < 0.01$.

9.3 Part 2: The Influence of *Bufeiyishen* Grain on Bronchial Lung Tissue Metalloprotease in Rats COPD Model

9.3.1 *Method*

(1) Experimental materials:

105 Wistar rats (Provided by Experimental Animal Center, Henan Medical University) of both sexes weighing 185–220 g. **Bacterial** *Klebsiella pneumoniae* (lot No.: 46114), provided by the National Institute for the Control of Pharmaceutical and Biological Products (NICPBP). Culturing and preservation of the bacteria was carried out followed routine procedures: the bacteria was cultured and preserved according to conventional methods of Bacteria Laboratory, Henan Provincial Medical Center, *K. pneumoniae* was diluted to 6×10^8 CFU/ml (confirmed by preliminary experiments) with sterile normal saline. **Smoked chamber** 300 L sealed plexiglass box. *Hongqiqu* brand filter cigarettes, Tar Content: 12 mg, Nicotine Content: 1.0 mg. *Bufeiyishen* Granule: Ibid manufacturer. *Yupingfeng* Granules (0.5 g/Granule) from Guangdong Otsuka Pharmacy Co., Ltd., Lot No.: 990905. Flumucil (600 mg/ tablet) from Zambon Group, Italy, Lot No.: 03D03/01.

(2) Experimental methods:

- Establishing stable COPD model
  Wistar rats were randomly divided into stable model group and control group. *K. pneumoniae* (6×10^8 CFU/ml) were injected into COPD model rats through nasal cavity. The injections lasted for eight weeks, with five days interval between two injections.

Intranasal injection: Administered 0.1 ml culture medium or bacteria using a 1 ml sterile syringe (with #5.5 needle, tightly connected to plastic tube) into the nares, injected when rats inhaled. The animals were initially exposed to eight cigarettes each time in weeks one and two, and the dose was increased to 15 cigarettes each time in week three to week 15. Cigarette smoke was delivered into the smoked chamber through a tube. Each smoke exposure lasted for 30 min, with a three hours resting period between cigarettes, three times per day.

- Establishing acute exacerbation of COPD animal model.

Following the establishment of COPD stable model, the model was verified after week 12, confirming that the model meet the COPD pathological features. Based on COPD stable model, the rats were intranasal injected with a high dose (0.3 ml) of *K. pneumoniae* (6×10^{12} CFU/ml, confirmed by preliminary experiments) from day four of week 13, twice a day, COPD acute exacerbation model was established four days after injection. In ten randomly chosen rats, 1 ml of blood from carotid artery was collected and heparinized, and then sealed in syringe. Tests of experimental rats showed a decrease in partial pressure of oxygen in arterial blood (PaO_2) and an increase in partial pressure of carbon dioxide in arterial blood ($PaCO_2$). Animals exhibited symptoms including gasping, dyspnea, wheezing rale, decreasing in exercise capacity.

- Grouping and processing.

Wistar rats were randomized into seven groups according the body weight, control group, stable COPD animal model group (stable model group), acute exacerbation of COPD animal model group (acute exacerbation model group), high-dose *Bufeiyishen* Grain group (high-dose group), low-dose *Bufeiyishen* Granule group (low-dose group), Flumucil group and *Yupingfeng* group, with 15 rats in each group. From week eight, the control group and groups were gastrically perfused of saline solution two times per day, whereas the high-dose group, low-dose group, *FuLuShi* group and *Yupingfeng* group were perfused with *Bufeiyishen* Grain ($28 \text{ g} \cdot \text{Kg}^{-1} \cdot \text{d}^1$), *Bufeiyishen* Granule ($12.6 \text{ g} \cdot \text{Kg}^{-1} \cdot \text{d}^{-1}$), Flumucil ($2.3 \text{ mg} \cdot \text{Kg}^{-1} \cdot \text{d}^{-1}$), *Yupingfeng* capsule ($0.482 \text{ g} \cdot \text{Kg}^{-1} \cdot \text{d}^{-1}$) respectively, two times per day. From day one of week 17, the acute exacerbation model group, high-dose group, low-dose group, Flumucil group, and *Yupingfeng* group were intranasally injected with a high dose (0.3 ml) of *K. pneumoniae* (6×10^{12} CFU/ml, confirmed by preliminary experiments) for three days, two times a day, then acute exacerbation was induced until day four of week 17, where sample collection was started.

(3) **Sample collection and processing:**
- Venous blood sample collection.
  Blood samples were obtained from vein for routine blood test at day one of week 17 before inducing the acute exacerbation model and day four of week 17 before the end of the experiment.
- Arterial blood sample collection.
  Blood was drawn from abdominal aorta and serum was prepared, arterial blood was heparinized and then sealed for future use. PaO_2 and $PaCO_2$ level in experimental rats were analyzed by Stat Profile 5 Blood Gas Analyzer.
- Bronchoalveolar lavage fluid (BALF).
  After taking of blood sample, cutting the neck skin, isolating the trachea and inserting a venous catheter, bronchi and alveolus were lavaged four times with 2–3 ml of saline solution, the recovery rate was around 70–80%. The recovered fluid was pooled and then centrifuged at 2000 rpm for 10 mins at 4, the supernatant was aliquoted and frozen ($-70°C$), and the pellet was used for cell counts.
- Left lung bronchial lavage.
  After lavage the lung was promptly fixed with formalin. Partial tissues of right middle lobe, upper lobe and inferior lobe were stored in liquid nitrogen for matrix metalloproteinase (MMPs) activity test. Right lung upper, middle and inferior lobe were fixed by formalin for immunohistochemistry and MMPs testing.
- Rats lung function tests.
  Rats were placed in the closed plethysmographical box which was connected to the sensor outside. While the animals were breathing, the ups and downs of thoracic cage altered the volume of plethysmographical box, changes of the volume were converted to electrical signals through pressure transducer and amplifier, the signals

were processed by computer and the respiration curves were displayed on the computer screen, then the respiratory rate, tidal volume (*Vt*), maximal voluntary ventilation (MMV), inspiratory resistance (*Ri*), expiratory resistance (Re) and compliance of lung (CL) were calculated after analyzing the graphs by associated software. The external pressure method was used: a "Y" shaped tube in between the tube and pressure transducer was connected, 8 ml air was pumped through a "Y" shaped tube to make deep inspiration and expiration in the animals, and checked the PEF and FEV0.3 levels, which reflected the condition of airflow destruction.

(4) Statistical analyses:
Statistical analyses were conducted using SPSS 11.0 for Windows. Quantitative data was tested for verification of normal distribution, data accorded with normal distribution was tested using one-way ANOVA, data that was not normally distributed was converted to be in accordance with the normal distribution or subjected to non-parametric test; $\alpha = 0.05$ (or $p < 0.05$) was taken as statistically significant. All values are expressed as average ($\overline{X}$) ± standard deviation (s).

9.3.2 *Results*

9.3.2.1 *Changes of leukocyte and neutrophil counts in blood*

(1) Leukocyte counts in peripheral blood (Table 9.2):
Before establishing acute exacerbation model, peripheral blood leukocyte counts in rats showed no obvious difference between groups ($p > 0.05$). Leukocyte counts were found to be higher in the acute exacerbation model group, high-dose group, low-dose group, *Yupingfeng* group, and Flumucil group than in the control group ($p < 0.01$) and stable model group ($p < 0.01$) at day four. Leukocyte counts were higher in the acute exacerbation model group, high-dose group, low-dose group, *Yupingfeng* group and Flumucil group at day four, compared to the counts before establishing the model ($p < 0.05$, $p < 0.01$).

Table 9.2. Changes of peripheral blood leukocyte counts $\times 10^{12}$ ($\bar{x} \pm s$, $n = 10$).

Group	16 weeks	16 weeks $+$ 4d
Control group	15.454 ± 3.581	15.897 ± 2.764
Stable model group	17.897 ± 4.565	17.341 ± 4.831
Acute exacerbation model group	17.860 ± 3.832	$28.144 \pm 6.531^{\#**}$
High-dose group	18.887 ± 4.241	$26.404 \pm 7.224^{\#*}$
Low-dose group	16.947 ± 4.354	$26.861 \pm 6.814^{\#**}$
Yupingfeng group	18.374 ± 4.125	$26.607 \pm 5.867^{\#**}$
FuLuShi group	18.877 ± 6.213	$27.458 \pm 5.642^{\#**}$

Compare to control group: $p < 0.05$, $p < 0.01$; compare to stable model group: #$p < 0.01$; compare to the values before establishing the model: *$p < 0.05$, **$p < 0.01$.

(2) Neutrophil counts in peripheral blood (Table 9.3):

Before establishment of the acute exacerbation model, peripheral blood neutrophil counts in rats showed no obvious difference between groups. Neutrophil counts were higher in acute exacerbation model group, high-dose group, low-dose group, *Yupingfeng* group and Flumucil group than the control group ($p < 0.01$) and stable model group ($p < 0.01$) after establishing the model. Leukocyte counts in the acute exacerbation model group, high-dose group, low-dose group, *Yupingfeng* group and Flumucil group were higher, compared to the counts before establishing the model ($p < 0.01$).

Table 9.3. Changes of peripheral blood neutrophil counts $\times 10^{12}$ ($\bar{x} \pm s$, $n = 10$).

Group	16 weeks	16 weeks + 4d
Control group	4.561 ± 0.881	4.658 ± 0.954
Stable model group	5.921 ± 1.472	5.426 ± 1.120
Acute exacerbation model group	5.964 ± 1.092	$9.984 \pm 2.021^{\#*}$
High-dose group	5.314 ± 1.091	$9.076 \pm 1.841^{\#*}$
Low-dose group	5.202 ± 1.082	$8.957 \pm 1.991^{\#*}$
Yupingfeng group	5.298 ± 1.069	$9.154 \pm 1.937^{\#*}$
FuLuShi group	5.378 ± 1.086	$9.174 \pm 1.699^{\#*}$

Compare to control group: $p < 0.05$, $p < 0.001$; compare to stable model group: #$p < 0.01$; compare to the values before establishing the model: *$p < 0.01$.

Table 9.4. Changes of leukocyte counts and neutrophil counts in BALF $\times 10^5$ ($\bar{x} \pm s$, $n = 10$).

Group	Leukocyte	Neutrophil
Control group	1.717 ± 0.342	0.141 ± 0.025
Stable model group	2.611 ± 0.524	$0.409 \pm 0.075^{\#}$
Acute exacerbation model group	$4.575 \pm 0.941^{\#}$	$1.531 \pm 0.414^{\#}$
High-dose group	$3.704 \pm 0.442^{\#\blacktriangle}$	$0.754 \pm 0.104^{\#\blacktriangle}$
Low-dose group	$3.817 \pm 0.508^{\#}$	$1.568 \pm 0.515^{\#}$
Yupingfeng group	$4.123 \pm 0.666^{\#}$	$1.439 \pm 0.481^{\#}$
FuLuShi group	$4.287 \pm 0.527^{\#}$	$1.389 \pm 0.550^{\#}$

Compare to control group: $p < 0.05$, $p < 0.01$; compare to stable model group: $\#p < 0.01$; compare to acute exacerbation model group: $\blacktriangle p < 0.05$.

9.3.2.2 *Changes of cell counts in BALF (Table 9.4)*

The acute exacerbation model group, stable model group, high-dose group, low-dose group, *Yupingfeng* group and Flumucil group showed obvious higher leukocyte counts and neutrophil counts in BALF than the control group ($p < 0.05$ or $p < 0.01$) and stable model group ($p < 0.01$). Leukocyte counts and neutrophil counts in BALF were found lower in the high-dose group than acute exacerbation model group ($p < 0.05$).

9.3.2.3 *Changes of lung function parameters (Table 9.5)*

The acute exacerbation model group, stable model group, high-dose group, low-dose group, *Yupingfeng* group and Flumucil group presented with obviously lower MVV, peak expiratory volume (PEF), $FEV_{0.3}/FVC\%$, compared to the control group ($p < 0.01$). Similarly, the acute exacerbation model group, high-dose group, low-dose group, *Yupingfeng* group and *FuLuShi* group had obvious lower MVV, PEF, $FEV_{0.3}/FVC\%$ than the stable model group ($p < 0.01$). MVV, PEF, $FEV_{0.3}/FVC\%$ in the high-dose group and low-dose group were obviously higher than in the acute exacerbation model group ($p < 0.05$).

Table 9.5. Changes of lung function parameters ($\bar{x} \pm s$, $n = 10$).

Group	MVV (ml)	PEF (ml/s)	$FEV_{0.3}/FVC$ %
Control group	137.9 ± 10.4	30.7 ± 2.9	84.2 ± 1.6
Stable model group	101.2 ± 8.1	21.7 ± 1.5	69.8 ± 2.9
Acute exacerbation model group	$81.1 \pm 5.7^{\#\#}$	$13.6 \pm 1.1^{\#\#}$	$54.9 \pm 4.0^{\#\#}$
High-dose group	$91.2 \pm 6.7^{\#\#\blacktriangle}$	$15.0 \pm 1.2^{\#\#\blacktriangle}$	$59.8 \pm 3.1^{\#\#\blacktriangle}$
Low-dose group	$86.4 \pm 5.8^{\#\#}$	$14.2 \pm 1.1^{\#\#}$	$56.6 \pm 5.0^{\#\#}$
Yupingfeng group	$83.6 \pm 5.5^{\#\#}$	$13.5 \pm 1.3^{\#\#}$	$56.9 \pm 6.8^{\#\#}$
FuLuShi group	$85.4 \pm 4.6^{\#\#}$	$14.1. \pm 1.7^{\#\#}$	$56.8 \pm 3.8^{\#\#}$

Compare to control group: $p < 0.01$; compare to stable model group: $\#p < 0.05$, $\#\#p < 0.01$; compare to acute exacerbation model group: $\blacktriangle p < 0.05$.

9.3.2.4 *Blood gas parameters (Table 9.6)*

The stable model group, acute exacerbation model group, high-dose group, low-dose group, *Yupingfeng* group and Flumucil group showed obviously lower PaO_2 levels than the control group ($p < 0.01$). PaO_2 levels in the acute exacerbation model group, high-dose group, low-dose group, and *Yupingfeng* group and Flumucil group were obviously lower than in the stable model group ($p < 0.05$), and PaO_2 levels in the high-dose group were higher, compared to acute exacerbation model group, *Yupingfeng* group and Flumucil group ($p < 0.01$).

Table 9.6. Changes of blood gas parameters ($\bar{x} \pm s$, $n = 10$).

Group	PaO_2(mmHg)	$PaCO_2$(mmHg)
Control group	91.765 ± 3.440	35.593 ± 3.396
Stable model group	67.579 ± 4.105	50.895 ± 7.652
Acute exacerbation model group	$46.109 \pm 5.679^{\#\#}$	$63.881 \pm 4.524^{\#\#}$
High-dose group	$56.681 \pm 4.682^{\#\#\blacktriangle\blacktriangle}$	$54.001 \pm 6.121^{\blacktriangle\blacktriangle}$
Low-dose group	$49.602 \pm 4.529^{\#\#}$	$61.964 \pm 5.519^{\#\#}$
Yupingfeng group	$49.904 \pm 5.031^{\#\#}$	$59.001 \pm 4.979^{\#\#}$
FuLuShi group	$45.989 \pm 5.798^{\#\#}$	$60.681 \pm 5.124^{\#\#}$

Compare to control group: $p < 0.05$, $p < 0.01$; compare to stable model group: $\#p < 0.05$, $\#\#p < 0.01$; compare to acute exacerbation model group: $\blacktriangle p < 0.05, \blacktriangle p < 0.01$.

9.3.2.5 *Changes of MMPs activity in lung tissue (Tables 9.7 and 9.8)*

Table 9.7 showed obvious higher 92 KD levels in the stable model group, acute exacerbation model group, high-dose group, low-dose group, *Yupingfeng* group and Flumucil group as compared to the control group ($p < 0.01$). Similarly, 82 KD levels were found to be higher ($p < 0.01$) in the stable model group, acute exacerbation model group, high-dose group, *Yupingfeng* group and Flumucil group. The high-dose group and low-dose group had both lower levels of 92 KD ($p < 0.01$) and 82 KD ($p < 0.01$) than acute exacerbation model group ($p < 0.01$).

Table 9.8 exhibited obvious higher 72 KD level in the stable model group, acute exacerbation model group, *Yupingfeng* group and Flumucil group as compared to the control group ($p < 0.01$). No obvious differences were observed between the high-dose group, low-dose group and stable model group ($p > 0.05$), but the high-dose group had lower levels of 72 KD than acute exacerbation model group ($p < 0.01$).

The stable model group, acute exacerbation model group, high-dose group, *Yupingfeng* group and Flumucil group had higher 62 KD levels than the control group ($p < 0.01$), whereas the levels were found to be lower in the high-dose group and low-dose group as compared to the acute exacerbation model group ($p < 0.05, p < 0.01$).

Table 9.7. Changes of MMP-9 in lung tissue of the rats ($\bar{x} \pm s$, $n = 10$).

Group	92 KD	82 KD
Control group	9.148 ± 3.701	0.967 ± 0.391
Stable model group	23.521 ± 5.812	2.513 ± 0.438
Acute exacerbation model group	53.235 ± 16.897	5.746 ± 1.018
High-dose group	$32.870 \pm 8.779^{\blacktriangle\blacktriangle}$	$2.584 \pm 0.928^{\blacktriangle\blacktriangle}$
Low-dose group	$34.423 \pm 8.310^{\blacktriangle\blacktriangle}$	$2.894 \pm 0.869^{\blacktriangle\blacktriangle}$
Yupingfeng group	49.173 ± 15.241	5.649 ± 0.995
FuLuShi group	50.915 ± 14.393	6.763 ± 1.293

(Enzyme unit U: A × mm²/10 μg) compare to control group: $p < 0.01$; compare to acute exacerbation model group: $\blacktriangle p < 0.05$, $\blacktriangle\blacktriangle p < 0.01$.

Table 9.8. Changes of MMP-2 in lung tissue of the rats ($\bar{x} \pm s$, $n = 10$).

Group	72 KD	62 KD
Control group	6.795 ± 4.915	2.297 ± 1.661
Stable model group	17.325 ± 4.528	5.862 ± 1.401
Acute exacerbation model group	45.591 ± 12.622	15.889 ± 2.581
High-dose group	35.984 ± 8.697▲▲	11.864 ± 2.843▲▲
Low-dose group	40.026 ± 7.765	12.861 ± 3.451▲
Yupingfeng group	40.365 ± 13.697	14.871 ± 3.579
FuLuShi group	41.122 ± 13.125	13.991 ± 2.912

(Enzyme unit U: $A \times mm^2/10\,\mu g$) compare to control group: $p < 0.01$; compare to acute exacerbation model group: ▲$p < 0.05$, ▲▲$p < 0.01$.

9.3.2.6 *Pathomorphological changes of lung*

The tracheal and bronchial were regular in the control group and there was no loss of cilia, but there were loss and reduction of the tracheal and bronchial cilia in the other groups, together with goblet cell hyperplasia. No degeneration of bronchial epithelial cells, no exudates in alveolar space, and no thickening of alveolar septum were observed. Obvious bronchial inflammatory cell infiltration, goblet cell hyperplasia, proliferation of smooth muscle, and loss of epithelium occurred in the stable model group. There were clear bronchiolar inflammatory cells infiltration, proliferation of smooth muscle, respiratory bronchiole narrowing and blocking; severe damage of bronchiolar epithelial cell, goblet cell hyperplasia and increase in lymphocyte and macrophages infiltration were also observed. Mucus occurred in respiratory bronchiolar lumen, and there was obvious bronchiolar wall smooth muscle cell and connective tissue hyperplasia, together with idiopathic pulmonary fibrosis. Surrounding areas of bronchioles, alveolar septum and alveolar space had clear inflammation; lymphocyte, plasmacyte and macrophage infiltration were augmented in alveolar septum, alveolar space was enlarged irregularly, focal alveolar septum destruction was also observed in the region, fusion of pulmonary alveolus caused emphysema. For the acute exacerbation model group, in addition to the changes in stable model group, bronchial mucosa hyperemia and edema, wide neutrophil infiltration in lumen and alveolar space, increase of mucus secretion, luminal plug formation, and regional field pulmonary consolidation were also observed. Comparing the Flumucil group and *Yupingfeng* group to the acute exacerbation model group, there was no significant decrease of inflammation. The high-dose group and low-dose group showed relative milder bronchial mucosa hyperemia and edema, there was neutrophil infiltration in lumen and alveolar space and elevated mucus secretion.

9.4 Discussion

9.4.1 *Effects of Bufeiyishen Granule to lung function and number of acute exacerbation in stable COPD*

Chronic obstructive pulmonary disease (COPD) is characterized by largely irreversible airflow obstruction; acute exacerbation can further decrease lung function, even patient morality. Our clinical study presented obvious increases of FEV1.0, MMEF, PEF and FEV1.01% in stable COPD patients two months after taking *Bufeiyishen* Grain, indicating the airflow improving function of *Bufeiyishen* Grain. The numbers of acute exacerbation were decreased significantly in the two groups after treatment ($p < 0.01$), with better effects in the treatment group than the control group ($p < 0.01$).

Animal experiments in this study showed obvious lower level of MVV, PEF, $FEV1.0_{0.3}/FVC\%$ in acute exacerbation model group, stable model group, low-dose group as compared to control group; with the result of obvious higher level of these parameters in the high-dose group than acute exacerbation model group, indicating that *Bufeiyishen* Grain could improve the airflow.

9.4.2 *The establishment of COPD animal model by composite factors*

Methods for developing animal model in recent COPD study include intratracheal injection of trypsin, cigarette smoke-inducing, SO_2 inhalation, and bacterial infection-induction (Snider *et al.*, 1986; Wright and Churg, 1990; Xu *et al.*, 2000; Xu *et al.*, 1999). All these models are only stable models which reflect a certain factor of the disease; an acute exacerbation model is lacking. In this research, we combined cigarette smoking and bacterial infection methods to make the stable COPD animal model, and developed an acute exacerbation of COPD animal model by further intranasal injection of high dose bacteria. The establishment of the models was successful, revealed by factors like lung function, pathological features, bronchial BALF inflammatory cell, etc.

Testing of lung function in stable COPD rats showed obvious lower Vt, PEF and higher IP as compared to control group, indicating airflow obstruction in airway. Leukocyte counts, neutrophil counts, macrophages were found to be obviously higher in BALF of the stable COPD rats, suggesting airway of the model rats appeared to have neutrophil and macrophage mediated inflammatory response; the COPD model rats exhibited gasping, dyspnea, which resembled symptoms in human COPD. Acute exacerbation model rats had obviously decreased PaO_2 levels and increased $PaCO_2$ levels, as compared to the stable model group; lung function tests showed obvious lower Vt, PEF and higher IP in the acute exacerbation model group, indicating further obstruction of airflow. Peripheral blood leukocyte, neutrophil counts were increased significantly in acute exacerbation model group compared to the stable model group; similar increases of leukocyte counts, neutrophil counts and macrophages were observed in the acute exacerbation model BALF, suggesting that the model rats airway has mainly neutrophil and macrophage mediated inflammatory response; worsening gasping and dyspnea in model rats were similar to human COPD acute exacerbation symptoms. Observation of pathological features in stable model group showed clear bronchial and bronchiolar inflammatory cells infiltration, goblet cell hyperplasia, proliferation of smooth muscle, loss of epithelium, severe damage of bronchiolar epithelial cell, with idiopathic pulmonary fibrosis. Surrounding areas of bronchioles, alveolar septum and alveolar space developed clear inflammation; lymphocyte, plasmacyte and macrophages infiltration were augmented in alveolar septum; alveolar space was enlarged irregularly. The acute exacerbation model group rats exhibited bronchial mucosa hyperemia and edema, respiratory bronchiole narrowing and blocking, goblet cell hyperplasia, widely neutrophil infiltration in lumen and alveolar space, increasing of mucus secretion, luminal plug formation, and regional field pulmonary consolidation. There was also obvious bronchiolar wall smooth muscle cell and connective tissue hyperplasia, clear idiopathic pulmonary fibrosis, irregular enlargement of alveolar space, emphysema, increasing of neutrophil infiltration in surrounding areas of bronchioles and alveolar septum.

9.4.3 *The influence of Bufeiyishen Granule to MMPs in COPD*

In physiological conditions, the lung extracellular matrix (ECM) is in a dynamic balance of synthesis and degradation, where the release of protease or decreasing of antiprotease synthesis can lead to ECM degradation. The balance between matrix metalloproteinase-9 (MMP-9) and tissue inhibitor of matrix metalloproteinase-1 (TIMP-1) is considered the symbol of dynamic balance of airway destruction and repair (Finlay *et al.*, 1997; Lim *et al.*, 2000) This research showed that the smoking and infection-induced COPD model having increased levels of lung tissue MMP-2, MMP-9 and TIMP-1 level in immunohistochemistry, elevated levels of mRNA and protein expression of MMP-2, MMP-9 and TIMP-1, and also the activity of MMP-2, MMP-9; in the bacterial infection-induced COPD acute exacerbation, mRNA and protein expression of MMP-2, MMP-9 and TIMP-1 was enhanced significantly, together with the activity of MMP-2, MMP-9. All the observations indicated that in stable COPD, cigarette smoke and bacterial infection continuously stimulated alveolar and bronchial epithelial cell, fibroblast, etc., thus increasing the synthesis of MMP-9, MMP-2; enhancing mRNA and protein expression of TIMP-1, together with the elevation of type I, III and IV collagens and LN expression which was positively correlated with MMP-9, MMP-2. In bacterial infection-induced COPD acute exacerbation, signal transduction pathways of MMP-9, MMP-2 were activated, leading to the activation of MMP-9 and MMP-2, and then degradation of ECM; lung ECM destruction made it easier for inflammatory cells like lymphocyte and macrophages to enter the alveolar space, further releasing the inflammatory mediators to cause lung injuries in COPD, and hence promoting disease progression (Vlahovic *et al.*, 1999). The present study exhibited obvious lower level of 92 KD, 82 KD MMP-9 and 72 KD, 62 KD MMP-2, together with less mRNA and protein expression of MMP-2, MMP-9, and TIMP-1 in the high-dose group and low-dose group, as compared to the acute exacerbation model group. The results suggested the *Bufeiyishen* Grain was able to suppress the synthesis and activation of lung MMP-9, MMP-2 in acute exacerbation of COPD.

9.5 Conclusions

(1) A stable COPD rats model was developed by composite methods with cigarette smoke and respiratory *Klebsiella pneumoniae* infection. In this model, lung function resembled the feature of airflow obstruction, and pathological features presented the characteristic of airway remodeling, in accordance with the clinical pathogenesis and pathological, physiological characteristics of COPD.

(2) Short-term, repeatedly, appropriate amount intranasal injection of *K. pneumoniae* could establish the acute exacerbation of COPD rats model, the features accorded with major pathological and physiological characteristics of clinical acute exacerbation of COPD.

(3) *Bufeiyishen* Granule could suppress the activation of bronchial lung tissue MMP-9, MMP-2 in acute exacerbation of COPD; and reduce the expression level of MMP-9 and MMP-2.

(4) *Bufeiyishen* Granule could improve lung ventilatory function in COPD stable patients with syndrome of deficiency of lung-kidney *qi*.

(5) *Bufeiyishen* Granule could reduce the numbers of acute exacerbation in stable COPD patients with syndrome of deficiency of lung-kidney *qi*.

References

Chronic Obstructive Pulmonary Disease Team, Chinese Society of Respiratory Diseases, Chinese Medicine Association. (2007) Guidance of diagnosis and treatment of chronic obstructive pulmonary diseases (2007 edition). *Chinese J. Tuberc. Respir. Dis.* **30**(1), 8–17.

Finlay, G.A., O'Driscoll, L.R., Russell, K.J., *et al.* (1997) Matrix metalloproteinase expression and production by alveolar macrophages in emphysema. *Am. J. Respir. Crit. Care Med.* **156**(1), 240–247.

Lim, S., Roche, N., Oliver, B.G., *et al.* (2000) Balance of matrix metalloprotease-9 and tissue inhibitor of metalloproteinase-1 from alveolar macrophages in cigarette smokers. Regulation by interlekuin-10. *Am. J. Respir. Crit. Care Med.* **162**, 1355–1360.

Skrepnek, G.H., Skrepnek, S.V., *et al.* (2004) Epidemiology, clinical and economic burden, and natural history of chronic obstructive pulmonary disease and asthma. *Am. J. Manag. Care* **10**(5 Suppl), S129–138S.

Snider, G.L, Lucey, E.C. and Stone P.J. (1986) Animal models of emphysema. *Am. Rev. Respir. Dis.* **133**, 149–169.

Vlahovic, G., Russell, M.L., Mercer, R.R., *et al.* (1999) Cellular and connective tissue changes in alveolar septal walls in emphysema. *Am. J. Respir. Crit. Care Med.* **160**(6), 2086–2092.

Wright, J.L and Churg A. (1990) Cigrette smoke causes physiologic and morphologic changes of emphyse-ma in the guinea pig. *Am. Rev. Respir. Emphysema Dis.* 142, 1422–1428.

Xu, J.Y., *et al.*, (2000) Establishment of rat models of chronic obstructive pulmonary disease. *Chinese J. Pathophysiol.* **16**, 383–384.

Xu, H., Xiong M., Huang Q.H., *et al.* (1999) Induction of chronic obstructive pulmonary disease by bacterial infection. *Chinese J. Tuberc. Respir. Dis.* **22**, 739–742.

Chapter 10

Dental Disease in the Elderly — From an Integrated Medical Perspective

Sim-Kim Cheng

Abstract

Dental diseases in the elderly are usually chronic and often complicated by general illness and medications. An alternate approach to study geriatric dental disease is proposed. Relating oral diseases to systemic functional systems with TCM theory provide a more holistic view of both local and general pathological factors. Cross-referring TCM theory with modern research show evidence that dental diseases are in close association with general condition. Saliva is found to be an importance interface between systemic functions and oral environment. It can serves as an indicator or diagnostic aid for many systemic conditions.

Keywords: Geriatric Dentistry; Saliva; Dental Diseases; Autoimmune Diseases; Functional Diseases; Organ System; Oral Homeostasis; TCM Oral Medicine; Etiology of Oral Diseases.

10.1 Introduction

As the aging population of the world is increasing, geriatric medicine becomes more important for the healthcare profession. The elderly will become the dentist's major group of patients in the future. The causes of dental diseases are diverse and complicated. They ranges from simple physical trauma, microbial infection, altered immune responses, psychological disturbances to deteriorating natural environment. In the elderly, the causes of dental problems are frequently complicated by increasing underlying systemic medical condition and protracted use of drugs. The prevalent dental diseases in the elderly are coronary dental caries, periodontal disease and diseases of mucous membrane. These classification and nomenclatures of diseases (in western medicine) are usually based on structural changes. But the dental problems in the elderly involves not only structural defects but also functional deterioration. Modern dentistry has advanced tremendously in the last few decades such that restoration and replacement of oral tissue are usually successful, but restoration does not necessarily bring about reinstatement of full function, and functional disorder remains a challenge to the dentists. TCM, which is basically a functional medicine, can be utilized to complement the shortfall of western medicine.

10.2 Nature of Dental Diseases in the Elderly

The nature of dental diseases in elderly can be classified arbitrarily into two categories:

(1) structural defects, which includes loss of oral tissue due to long usage, attrition and diseases; and
(2) functional changes, which could be due to degeneration characterized by decline in regenerative capacity.

These two categories are interrelated and mutually affecting each other: structural defect causes lost or weakening of functions. Dysfunction can also leads to structural changes. Many functional disorders are due to two related factors: i.e. aging and underlying systemic diseases, which tend to increase or become more severe with aging. Structural defects can usually be rectified and the related function restored. Functional deteriorations are usually chronic and reinstatement is sometime difficult if not impossible. This is mainly due to the decline of regenerative ability, which is closely associated with aging and systemic diseases.

Examples of degeneration includes qualitative and quantitative changes of saliva, deteriorating regeneration ability, altered immune response and atrophic changes of oral tissue. Retarded cognition capability and depression are another two common problems among the elderly. Dental care for the elderly therefore not only involves repairing of structural defects but also restoring of function. An alternate set of theory and method is required to study functional disorder as western medicine usually focuses more on structural diseases.

10.3 TCM View on Dental Diseases

TCM regards the oral cavity as an integrated part of the body. The TCM's taxonomy of the body is base on complex structures rather than anatomical structures. The complex structures which are called organ systems (*zangfu* 臟腑) are composed of three different types of structures, namely: (1) spatial structure, (2) temporal structure, and (3) functional structure which is the basic and major component. For example, the organ system called *xin* (heart) is composed of three components: (1) the spatial structure is the anatomical heart and part of the central nervous system; (2) the functional structure governs blood circulation and dominates the mental activities; and (3) the temporal structure means the functions of *xin* can vary from time to time. Modern research had shown that the organ system *shen* (kidney system) is related structurally to the kidney organ as well as the hypothalamus, the pituitary gland and other endocrine organs. Its functions involve waste excretion, reproduction and hormonal activities. Various functions prevail at different time (Ref. 1). This method of categorization enables us to view the body beyond its physical structures and observe it from a functional aspect. Coordination of structures forms function which can be considered as the expression of interrelationships among structures. In addition to structural defects, changes in inter-relationship will lead to disparity in function. Phenomena which cannot be explained in terms of structural changes alone can now be elucidated through studying of the irregularity in their inter-relationships (Ref. 2).

The oral cavity is connected to the organ systems through networks of meridians. The meridians act as transportation pathway for material, energy and information. They forms an important part of the network of interrelationships by linking all superficies, orifices, limbs and joints to the internal organ system (*zangfu* 臟腑). Diseases can be transmitted from the superficies to the internal organ systems through the meridians. Disorder of these systems can also be reflected on the superficies including the oral cavity. Oral diseases are considered as the external manifestations of systemic conditions in TCM. Therefore, the oral cavity is in fact a window which can showcase many systemic disorders.

The elderly has two common systemic disorders: (1) deficiency of *qi* and blood, and (2) flagging organ systems. These two deteriorations are the main cause of many geriatric illnesses. These systemic conditions could be presented in the oral cavity as more severed periodontal diseases, diseases of the oral mucosa or other autoimmune conditions.

10.4 Oral Diseases as Manifestations of Systemic Disorders

(1) *Xin* (heart system) and oral condition.

Xin open into the tongue. The branch of hand *taiyin* heart meridian is connected to the body of the tongue. The color of the tongue, especially its tip serves as an indicator for the functional state of *xin*. Oral ulceration can be due to flaring up of heart fire. Depletion of heart *yin* causes dry mouth.

(2) *Pi* (spleen system) and oral condition.

Pi open into the mouth. The foot *taiyin* spleen meridian spreads to the base of tongue after passing through its body. Saliva is related to *pi*. Deficiency of *pi* causes uncontrolled salivation and drooling which could increase occurrence of angular cheilitis. Coating of the tongue can review the functional state of *pi*. Deficiency of *pi qi* shows swollen, light color, moldy mucous membrane with bleeding and recessed gums. A dry mouth, fragile, hyperaemic and slightly swollen mucous membrane can be seen in simultaneous deficiency of *xin* and *pi*. If heat is accumulated in both systems, there would be erosion of the mucous membrane with swollen and bleeding gum.

(3) *Wei* (stomach system) and oral condition.

The gum is called the capillaries of *wei* in TCM. The stomach meridian is connected to the large intestine meridian. The two meridians are distributed on the mandible and maxilla. Dysfunction of either system can lead to oral diseases. Trigeminal neuralgia is often associates with hyperfunction of the stomach or large intestine system. Stomach fire could be presented as hyperemic, suppurative swollen gum, red swollen cheek, ulceration, dry mouth, sticky saliva and is sometime accompanied with halitosis. Acute gingivitis and periodontitis are two common dental infections that related to *wei* fire. If damp heat attacks *pi* and *wei*, the saliva would become sticky with sweet taste in the mouth. Oral ulceration could be rampant. *Yin* deficiency of both systems results in dry mouth and lips, red dry tongue with peeled coating.

(4) *Shen* (kidney system) and oral condition

Spittle is the fluid of *shen*. The meridian of foot *shaoyin shen* meridian send branches upwards along the throat to the lateral sides of the base of

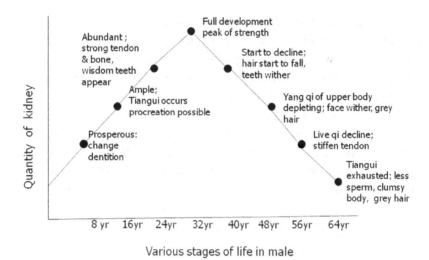

Fig. 10.1. Quantity of Kidney *qi* at various life stages in males.

tongue. Teeth are considered as the tip of the bone which is governed by the kidney system. The kidney is the most important organ system associated with growth, development and aging of the body.

《黄帝内经》 *The Yellow Emperor Canon of Internal Medicine* had illustrated that the growth, development and aging of the body is followed closely with the increase, abundance and decline of *shen qi* (kidney *qi*). At the age of 40, the kidney *qi* starts to decline and teeth begin to wither (see above illustration). TCM asserts that bone is governed by the kidney system. The growth of bone relies on the kidney essence and *qi*. The bone and teeth loses its strength as age increases. Modern research had confirmed that the number of osteoblasts decreases as the bone surface area and volume decrease with aging (Burkhardt *et al.*, 1987) (Ref. 3). Resorption of alveolar bone occur after loss of teeth. Imbalance of osteoclast and osteoblast activity aggravates such resorption. The symptoms of kidney *yin* deficiency include dry, red and cracked lower lip, mobile teeth with dull pain, hyperemic and infected gum with exudates. The mucous membrane would be thin, pale and degenerating. Oral ulceration if any would be less swollen and hyperemic. The affected area would be limited. In the case of deficiency of kidney *yang*, the color of the membrane would be light. The gum is generally thin and light in color or slightly swollen. Root exposure and erosion of periodontal bone are common. The teeth would appear dry and dull. Incoordination of heart and kidney systems show red, painful and cracked tongue with less coating. The teeth would be weak on occlusion and gums are receding. Kidney deficiency is one of the main causes of periodontal diseases in the elderly.

(5) *Gan* (liver system) and oral condition

Foot *jueyin* meridian of liver send branches to the tongue. Another branch descends from infraorbital margin to spread across the buccal mucosa and encircle the inner surface of the lips. Stagnation of liver *qi* can cause cysts, hard lumps or tumors on the tongue, cheek or gum. Stirring of internal wind generated from liver heat can results in atrophic tongue, deviated tongue, tremor of the tongue or aphasia. Flaring up of liver fire can be manifested as a bitter or sour taste in the mouth, oral facial pain or swollen gum.

The above TCM interpretations of oral conditions are based on functional perspective. The functional changes of the organ systems are the main mechanism used in explaining the pathology of the oral conditions. TCM asserts that instead of structural changes, it is the incoordinated actions of internal systemic structures that disrupt the functions and subsequently leads to changes of oral structures.

10.5 Oral Diseases of Unknown Etiology

Many oral diseases are autoimmune in nature with etiology unknown to western medicine. Diseases of oral mucous membrane are a group of diseases that is more prevalent in older patients. Autoimmune diseases are basically functional disorder in nature which can not be explained solely in terms of structural changes. An entirely different approach is required to understand and treat them. TCM opens up a new perspective through an alternate taxonomy with different methodology. It elucidates the occurrence of these diseases through a functional perspective that these diseases are the consequences of functional disturbances of some organ systems.

For example: recurrent aphthous ulcer, based on its nature, can be classified into excess or deficient type. The excess type could be due to accumulated heat or fire either in *pi* (spleen system), *wei* (stomach system), *gan* (liver system) or *xin* (heart system). The consequential ulceration is usually more painful and hyperemic. The deficient type of ulcer is usually less painful and hyperemic. They could be *due* to deficiency of either *pi yang*, *shen yang* or *pi qi*. The ulceration is the consequences of hyper-or hypo-function of the organ systems. Other diseases of unknown etiology can also be elucidated through identification of organ system with functional disorder.

Since all organ systems are inter-related, the internal environment of oral cavity is also closely associated with all organ systems and the essentials operating material of the body (*qi*, blood, body fluid). All of these have great effect on the oral environment. Recent study on saliva helps to explain how systemic condition can affect the oral environment.

10.6 Saliva as an Interface for Oral Homeostasis

Western medicine asserts that a homeostatic environment of oral cavity is vital for prevention of oral diseases. Oral ecologist maintains that the dynamic ecological balance (1) among the oral microorganisms, and (2) between the microflora and the host are both important in keeping the homeostasis of oral cavity. Saliva is the key substance that plays a great role in maintaining the homeostatic oral environment which is achieved by collaboration of multiple structural and functional systems. The nervous system, circulatory system, skeletal-muscular system, endocrine system, oral microflora and saliva are all involved in this multiple coordination. Saliva is the catalytic interface for many biological interactions. It is the common space for microorganisms to intermingle, compete, or collaborate. It also provides a venue for the body immune system to respond to various microorganisms. The temperature, pH value, viscosity, constituents and flow rate of the saliva readily affect the oral ecology system. The oral ecologists hold that it is the imbalance of the symbiotic relationship among the various microorganisms or displacement of certain microorganism from its usual habitat that cause infection. The composition of the saliva includes mucin, ammonia, urea, nitrites, minerals, protein, immunoglobulin and enzymes, etc. These substances coordinate to form the various functions of saliva, e.g. cleansing, lubrication, digestion, repair and defense, etc. Changes in quantity and quality of saliva cause disturbance to the normal flora of the oral cavity. The reduced flow of saliva decreases the cleaning effect and thus encourages plaque accumulation, which increases chances of dental caries and periodontal diseases. The mucin content of the saliva provides lubrication to protect the oral mucosa from abrasion during mastication. Enzymes and immunoglobulin helps forming the oral immune system. The synergistic actions of these contents provide multiple defense functions of the host. These protections collapse when the salivary flow rate drops to a certain level (Tenovuo, 1998). Primary digestion of food takes place in the mouth by the action of various digestive enzymes. Any alteration in the properties of the saliva can affects the integrity of oral tissue, their regeneration, the oral immune system and maintenance of normal masticatory functions. Sreebny (2000) had shown that unstimulated flow of saliva decreases with aging. Queiroz *et al.* (2002) also shows that stress and anxiety readily reduces the flow rate of saliva. 郝巧英 *et al.* discovered that stressful occupation decreases sIgA in saliva (Ref. 7).

The constituents of saliva are dependent on blood supply to the salivary gland. The blood supplied in turn varies with multiple factors which are related to many anatomical (organs) and functional systems of the body. Since the organ systems are connected to the oral cavity through the meridians, changes in these organ systems can readily affect the quality and quantity of the saliva.

10.7 Effect of Organ Systems on Saliva

TCM classifies saliva into two types: the thinner or less viscous type of saliva is called drool (涎). The thicker or more viscous type is called spittle (唾). This is consistent with the fact that saliva secreted from different salivary glands do varies in viscosity and contents. Drool is controlled by *pi* (spleen system). Spittle is governed by *shen* (kidney system). *Pi* or *shen* disorder can be detected in qualitative or quantitative changes of the saliva. For example, hypofunction of *pi* (*pi* deficiency) can be manifested as overflow of saliva from the mouth. The drooling causes persistent wetness at angle of the mouth which often leads to cheilitis. Deficiency of kidney *yin* can cause dry mouth with reduced salivary flow. Taste changes take place in disorders of various organ systems. For example: a sweet taste in the mouth could mean damp heat invasion. Heat in *xin* (heart), *gan* (liver) or *dan* (gall bladder) cause bitter taste. Deficiency of *shen* (kidney) causes a salty taste in the mouth.

Many TCM classics had reported on the effects of diseases on salivary flow. When cross-referring these documents with the modern research findings, it is reasonable to deduce that functions of organ systems affect saliva by altering its contents as well as its flow rate.

陈德珍 *et al.* found lower flow rate of saliva in patients with *yin* deficiency of *pi* (spleen) or *shen* (kidney). (Ref. 8) 李碧 *et al.* had shown that in patient with deficiency of *pi* and *shen* or deficiency of *qi* and blood, there is significant drop in protein content in their saliva. They also discovered that the salivary urea and potassium content is directly proportional to their blood content in patient with kidney dysfunction. (Ref. 9). Recent research had pointed out that saliva can be used as a non-invasive tool for diagnosis of various systemic diseases (Ref. 10).

The effect of organ systems on oral health can be summarized as the following:

From the below research in saliva, it is conceivable that the quantity and quality of saliva are both vital to the maintenance of oral health. Any measure that can maintain the normal flow and constituents of saliva definitely helps in keeping good oral health. Normal flow rate and properties of saliva rely on proper functioning of the various systems in the body. Therefore, in addition to keep good dental hygiene and regular check-ups, preventive measures should be extended to ensuring the proper function of other physiological systems.

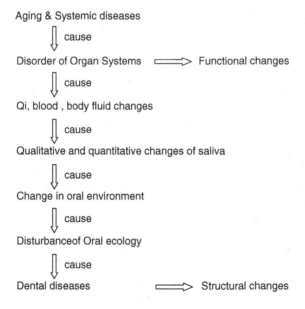

10.8 Conclusion

Aging causes declination of physiological functions. These deteriorations are usually aggravated by the underlying systemic diseases and reduced ability to recover. TCM not only provides an alternate view in explaining the etiology and pathology of dental diseases, it also made available many avenues for treatment of functional diseases. Hippocrates had said that diseases always started and remain as general disorder. TCM holds the same view that dental diseases are manifestation of general condition. Both local and general conditions should be taken into consideration in treatment and prevention of dental diseases in the elderly. The oral condition could also be useful as an indicative of underlying systemic disorder. Modern medicine had already made use of saliva as medium for non-invasive investigation for many diseases. Modern dentistry is excellent at restoring structural defects and TCM should be employed to regulate the functional changes. Dental treatment would be more accomplished with integration of TCM and modern dentistry.

References

Burkhardt, R., Kettner, G., Bihm, W. *et al.* (1987) Changes in trabecular bone, haematopoiesis and bone marrow vessels in aplastic anemia, primary osteoporosis, and old age: A comparative histomorhometric study. *Bone* **8**, 157–164.

Chen D.Z., *et al.* (1996) Detection of salivary lysozyme and analysis of salivary flow speed in patients with *yin* deficiency of *pi* and *shen*. *Jiang Shu Zhong Yi* **17**(11), 42.

Hao Q.Y., *et al.* (2002) Relationship between saliva immunoglobulin A and occupational stress in nurses. *Res. Nurs. Care* **16**(4), 207.

Herenia, P.L. (2002) Salivary markers of systemic disease: Nonivasive diagnosis of disease and monitoring of general health. *J. Can. Den. Assoc.* **68**(3), 170.

Li, B., Qing, J.H., *et al.* (1986) Research of "Fluid and blood have the same origin" and "Spittle as expression of *shen*". *J. Shandong Med. Sch.* **10**(3), 23.

Queiro, C.S. *et al.* (2002) Relationship between stressful situation, salivary flow rate and oral volatile sulfur-containing compounds. *Eur. J. Oral. Sci.* **110**(5), 337.

Shen, Z.Y. (1988) *The Modern Research in TCM Theory.* Jiangshu Scientific Press, pp. 3–12 [in Chinese].

Sreebny, L.M. (2000) Saliva in health and diseases: An appraisal and update. *Int. Den. J.* **50**, 140–161.

Tenovuo, J. (1998) Antimicrobial function of human saliva — How important is it for oral health? *Acta. Odontal. Scand.* **56**(5), 250–256.

Zhu, S.N. and Huang, T.K. (2002) *TCM System Theory and System Engineering.* China TCM Publishing House, pp. 259–261 [in Chinese].

Chapter 11

Natural Healing in Chinese Medicine: Qi Gong and Tai Chi

Ping-Chung Leung

Abstract

Exercises involving stretching and control breathing are among the most important measures for the maintenance of health and natural healing according to the ancient *Chinese Classic on Medicine*. Meditation is another essential component in the pursuit of health.

Qi Gong and *Tai Chi* are the most common body training practices requiring the tripartite combination of stretching, controlled breathing and meditation. The physiological basis of the practices are described in this chapter. While carefully planned clinical investigations have been performed to show the physiological benefits of *Qi Gong* and *Tai Chi,* the perfect scientific explanations are still remote. This tripartite combination of stretching, control breathing and meditation can help stimulate infrequent neurological activities and its versatility will encourage this practice in all health-conscious individuals.

Keywords: Wellness; Natural Healing Qi Gong; Tai Chi.

11.1 Introduction

Natural Healing as a means to promote health and treating diseases is becoming popular in Europe and America. If Natural Healing refers to the maintenance of Health without specific drug or other means of treatment, it has long existed in China. For thousands of years, a unique system of health promotion using natural means, *viz.* food, life style and exercises, has developed, matured and has been widely practiced in China. 'Natural

Healing' might not be the best term to describe this system of health promotion but it is difficult to create more appropriate terminologies. One direct translation of this system of health promotion, Young-Shung (養生), could be the maintenance or promotion of wellness. Wellness refers to the physical, physiological, and psycho-social aspects of living, through careful self-endeavours of food intake, life styles and exercises (Wang, 2008; Huang, 2009).

Joseph Needham pointed out in his great work on *History of Science and Technology in China*, that the system of self-performed health maintenance in Ancient China never existed anywhere else in the world. Indeed, Natural Healing (we still use this terminology in view of the lack of appropriate substitute for a general understanding) in Chinese Medicine exists as a complete system with a strong philosophical basis, involves careful professional, i.e. medical conceptualization, defines complicated methodologies of practice, and in recent years, commands organized social networks for its promotion (Wang, 2007; Lic, 2003).

11.2 Philosophical Background

Natural Healing is strongly linked to the philosophy of Taoism. The philosopher Zuangtze 莊子 used a colourful story to illustrate his thoughts about the clever utilization of a tool which reflected to the living of one's life. An experienced butcher has used his cutting knife for 19 years and found that it remained sharp. Of course, the butcher skillfully cut through the joints of the animals to get the meat out and never hit his knife against the hard bones. Human life could remain colourful and pleasant only if one avoids the tough currents and learns about the skill to maintain one's best performance.

Another Taoist, Laotze, stressed about the importance of "plainness and laxity", i.e. a state of utter mental relaxation away from worldly pursues, as a means to longevity.

Although Taoists probably have given the most solid input to the philosophical basis of Natural Healing in China, the system of health maintenance has been influenced by other philosophical schools. At the very beginning, spiritual dancing which was linked with superstitious spiritual worship to get rid of misfortunes, initiated certain forms of exercises which evolved through superstition to health purposes. Then when Confucians talked about celestial observations, meteorology, climate changes and their influences on human activities, health was brought to a level of interaction between the Human and Heavenly Divine. All these Taoist and Confucian input must be responsible for the meditation aspect of Natural Healing in China. Buddhism came to China later during the Tang period. Buddhists' practice of meditation with special requirements on the sitting posture then supplied additional influence in the development of Natural Healing (Ji, 1994a, 1994b).

11.3 Concepts of Natural Healing

One of the mostly emphasized area of Health in the earliest classic of Chinese Medicine, Ne-jing, is Natural Healing. Natural Healing — maintaining a perfect state of physical and physiological survival, as well as a harmonious state of psychosocial well-being, is considered the goal of Health and longevity.

The overall concept involves the harmony between *yin* and *yang*; harmony between physique and psychosocial state; balanced nutrition, balanced exercises and recreation. The concept of *qi* is most important for Natural Healing. When *qi* remains healthy, abnormal physiological processes will not happen. *Qi* is the fundamental basis of survival, viability and vitality. *Qi* controls activities, changes and development. *Qi* has a direct form of respiration when air is inhaled through the nose to the lungs, thence, distributed throughout the body, along the meridians. *Qi* perpetuates on its own but needs continuous sustenance and reinforcement to maintain healthy development. Sustenance and reinforcement depends on repeated input of nutritional support and special exercises. *Qi* is not only the visible process of respiration which forms only the fundamental basis, *Qi* it is also a state of physiological harmony expressed as perfect survival and good living. *Qi* is at the same time an inner feeling of internal balance, well-being and capability (Ji, 1994c; 1994d; 1994e).

Qi does not exist alone. *Qi* co-exists with two other special states: which, in modern terms, could be understood as a state of balanced secretion (精 Jing) and a state of spiritual esteem (神 Shen). Detailed physiology is not known to the ancient healers, but they have good knowledge about visible secretions like saliva and secretions from the bowel and genitals. Their concept of "secretion" in fact has combined the exocrine and endocrine systems. Therefore, *jing* could be understood as a fundamental state of exocrine and endocrine balance. The state of spiritual esteem is easily interpreted today as psychosocial well-being (Si, 2006; Liang, 2005).

Natural Healing for Traditional Chinese Medicine, therefore, compiles the three components of physical, physiological and psychosocial harmony which are all interlinked. The ancient healers, through so many years of practice, have worked out varieties of means to help boostering the state of harmony.

11.4 Practice of Natural Healing

When Natural Healing is discussed, either under the popular European or American concept of today, or is considered with a modern Chinese Medicine context, it is commonly taken as activities related with treatment of a straight forward disease entity or activities arranged for rehabilitation. In reality, Natural Healing in Chinese Medicine has a much broader concept, which covers maintenance of health, wellness and prevention of falling sick. The perspective has been pushed to such an extreme as is being expressed by the advocates who believe that those well experienced with the practice would die but their dead bodies would not decay.

The two best-known varieties of Natural Healing today are *Qi Gong* and *Tai Chi*; the former allows a lot of practitioner's modifications while the latter follows a rigid system of chained activities (Yi, 2007; Wang and Xiang, 2006).

11.5 *Qi Gong*

The promotion of Natural Healing requires disciplined practices that would help bringing harmony to the three important components, *viz. qi*, *jing* and *shen*.

11.5.1 *Stretching*

Historically, spiritual dancing could have been the very early practice of Natural Healing. Hence, stretching movements while adopting a variety of postures have become the most essential components of practice. Early imitation of the postures of different animals have later evolved into chains of movements copying animal activities. Later, still different groups of practitioners created their own system of activities and motions with different connotations and hawmarks. The uniform component of these different systems is that, all of them consist of stretching movements. As far as posture is concerned: some advocates natural postures like standing, sitting; modification like "Buddha sitting", half-kneeling, animal postures, etc.

11.5.2 *Respiratory control*

The practice of Natural Healing invariably included controlled breathing without which there will be little value of the stretching exercises. *Qi Gong* might have inaccurately been assumed that it deals with *qi* only. In fact, it is the sustenance and development of the *qi*, that requires simultaneous stretching, controlled respiration and meditation. It is believed that, with skilful control of breathing, *qi* is manipulated successfully, so that it not only circulates through the respiratory system, but, together with meditation, it reaches the different physiological systems to improve their metabolic state of balance.

Respiration is controlled so that the normal pattern is not followed. The recommended patterns include extra-long inspiration of extra-long expiration. Abdominal or diaphragmatic breathing is also practiced. While doing so, the pelvic diaphragm and anal sphincters are also squeezed at will.

So, respiratory control is executed simultaneously with the stretching movements in a smooth synchronized chain of activities under the individual's free will. It would be up to the individual to develop his/her own policy of training which could be amended from time to time (Yang, 2001; Won, 2004).

11.5.3 *Meditation*

Natural Healing aims at harmonizing physical, humoral and mental activities. Meditation is an indispensible component. The intersectional harmony must be promoted. The skilful practitioner attains a tranquility of the mind while stretching is being performed with controlled breathing. It must be understood that meditation requires the simultaneous support from stretching and breathing and vice versa. The apparently complicated system of movements in *Tai Chi* should not be hindering meditation. Rather, they provide a good initiating environment where the day to day mental pressure will not be felt. The material background for meditation is resting of the central nervous system. During the training, the intention is to give a good rest to the Central Nervous System: free it from motor and sensory burdens, (apart from the comforting limb movements) relieve it from complex memories, protect it from emotions and problem solving requirements. The assumption is: with this unchallenged mental state, a reorganization of the interacting neurological messages can take place, initiating a regional (neurological) establishment of harmony and a re-organized humoral state (Won, 2008; Chen, 1998).

11.6 *Tai Chi*

While all the three components (stretching, controlled breathing and meditation) are stressed and must be practiced in the training, different schools of promotion keen to initiate modifications would find the stretching part most versatile for change. *Tai Chi*, for instance, allows colorful dancing movements with varying speeds. The whole set of arrangements is established after thorough consideration of the meridians and sites of the acupoints.

Tai Chi requires a fully relaxed body. While the four limbs moves in semicircular and circular movements, the focus remains around the waist, which rotates left and right. The movements stimulate the 300 acupoints of the whole body in a orchestrated manner. The result is a concerted, systematic stimulation of the acupoints, each one of which is related to certain somatic or sympathetic functions. All *Tai Chi* practitioners are aware of the circulatory activations once the *Tai Chi* exercises continue for a while. Recent functional magnetic resonance investigation on brain function have also preliminary evidences to show that the stimulation of acupuncture points does elicit functional changes in different parts of the brain (Jones, 2001; Hsu, 1986).

In fact, the term '*Tai Chi*' is self-explanatory. Just imagine the Tai Chi symbol which is a round circular figure within which habours two fish symbols, that go along a clockwise chase after each other (see Symbol of *Tai Chi*). *Tai Chi*, therefore, signifies the natural law of the universe, which is possessing perfect harmony and balance. Followers should therefore obey the law of balance between light and heavy, slow and fast, weak and strong, keep a well controlled breathing, avoid jerky motions, over strenuous movements, etc. Movements of the left and right arms could be viewed as *yin* and *yang* forces. The aim is to maintain their balance. Every movement in *Tai Chi*, needs to be synchronized with respiration. The concerted contractions of the muscle groups requires gentle oxygen intake and then join together and converge into a state of *qi* (*chi*) establishment (Green and Blankshy, 1996; Chang and Wai, 1997).

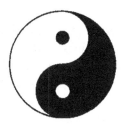

Symbol of Tai Chi太極圖

Students practicing *Tai Chi* are enlightened to be aware of four states of mind during the exercises

i) *A sense of central stability*
    Qi Gong principle states that *qi* starts with the nose, follows the midline trachea to the lungs, thence, follow the central line anteriorly along the midline to the umbilical region and at the central back to the upper lumbar region. Limb movements and body rotation is centered along this central pillar of Qi. With this concept in mind, *Tai Chi* performance is relaxed and accurate (Motoyama and Sunami, 1998).

    According to *Tai Chi* trainers, poor performances are related to a lack of understanding of controlled breathing, ignorance about training regulations, about the timing of adding strength, and failure to master the concept of *yin-yang* balance. Moreover, *Tai Chi* practice should not be over-energetic, otherwise, the pressure of quick achievement would affect relaxation and the need for meditation (Astsumi, 2007).

ii) *Awareness of the bony prominence*
    Bony prominences are all related to muscle attachments. Like the acupoints along the meridians, *Tai Chi* movements give them indirect stimulations. Intentional stretching relevant to the bony prominences have additional stimulation effects.
iii) *State of awareness relevant to the meridians*
    The practicing person should have a sound knowledge about the meridians and bear in mind the position of the acupoints during practice so that with a certain posture and a special movement, better stimulation can be given to the relevant acupoints.
iv) *State of tranquility*
    After sufficient time of practice Tai Chi gives the practitioner not only the usual relaxed state of calmness and pleasure, but an additional feeling of un-worldliness, sometimes described as a the state of euphoria experienced by a half-drunken individual. This pleasant state has been considered a measurement of achievement.

11.7 Clinical Research on *Qi Gong* and *Tai Chi*

Epidemiological surveys on people enjoying long life all showed that the common components for longevity include very good quality of life ever since they are born. Thus, the Okinawa study on centurians showed that these people living beyond 100 years had balanced healthy diets, plenty of exercise, and rich healthy social activities (Astsumi, 2007).

People practicing *Qi Gong* and *Tai Chi* realize that through gentle, disciplined exercises, they gain sustained muscular strength, general vitality and mental tranquility. They have reasons to believe that they become healthier and would live longer. People practicing *Tai Chi* and *Qi Gong* also claim that they do not fall sick and are not vulnerable to diseases. Those might be simple evidences supporting the Chinese Way of Natural Healing as being good for the prevention of diseases.

With the rising popularity of Natural Healing and the oriental influence on the perception of health, more and more people start to practice *Qi Gong* and *Tai Chi*. Academics and professionals have started to seriously look for the scientific basis of the Chinese Way of Natural Healing. Many reports on the clinical effects of *Qi Gong* and *Tai Chi* have appeared in the past decade. The following paragraphs attempt to give a glimpse of the research being done.

11.7.1 *Qi Gong*

In 2004, the Beijing Sport University conducted a clinical study on the effects of *Qi Gong* on the physical ability of a group of people aged from 50 to 70. Fifteen days of *Qi Gong* exercises were given to these people, after which their physical fitness was assessed and compared with their pre-study conditions. Parameters of assessment included basic musculoskeletal data like body weight, waist girdle, fat thickness, hand grip strength, leg strength and stance. Heart-lung fitness was also measured. The results showed that the basic physical state of the people under training, i.e. body weight, girdle and fat thickness etc did not change. The musculoskeletal activities, as were manifested by hand grip and leg strength improved. Balancing power also significantly improved. With regard to cardiopulmonary health: heart rate showed a steady state before and after the training period. Looking at the heart rate changes during the *Qi Gong* exercise, it was shown that the maximal, median and finishing heart rates all improved (lowered) towards the end of the training. This is a clear indication that the ability of the heart among this group of middle age and older age people to adapt to higher demand of physical activities improved with the *Qi Gong*. Respiratory function also improved after the period of training (Tsang and Chow, 2005).

In 2005, the Sports Institute of the Jiangxi University conducted a study on the cardiac function of 70 people, aged between 61 and 68, in response to a continuous training of *Qi Gong* of Stretching. The training lasted six months. A control group of 30 people was recruited, having quite similar body weights and heights. Cardiac function was assessed using high resolution ultrasonic equipment. The chosen parameters included

Table 11.1. Cardiac function before and after training (Du *et al.*, 2006).

	Control Group ($n = 31$)		Study Group ($n = 39$)	
	Before training	After six months' training	Before training	After six months' training
SV (ml)	57.94 ± 16.01	58.51 ± 16.99	55.72 ± 15.78	67.15 ± 13.67**#
VE (cm/s)	65.95 ± 19.95	66.30 ± 19.75	66.50 ± 18.24	75.05 ± 17.66**#
VA (cm/s)	84.36 ± 15.12	82.68 ± 14.10	83.02 ± 13.89	83.76 ± 15.21
VE-VA	-18.41 ± 23.98	-16.38 ± 24.68	-16.53 ± 25.96	-10.25 ± 23.32*

stroke volume (SV), early diastolic velocity (VE) and late diastolic velocity (VA).

The results in Table 11.1 showed better SV and VE in the trained group compared with the control group. VE-VA showed even a more convincing improvement (Du *et al.*, 2006).

On a related theme of cardiovascular function, changes in the serum fatty acid levels were studied before and after *Qi Gong* in the Talien Institute of Physical Training in 2008. For this study, 62 patients with high serum triglyceride levels were selected and randomly divided into the trial and control groups. The trial group was instructed for training on a scheme of 60 minutes per day for six months. Parameters of assessment included the molecular markers S1 CAM-1, SVCAM-1, Ps, Fig, TG, TC, LDL-C and HDL-C levels. After six months of *Qi Gong* exercises, HDL-C was higher in the study group while all the other markers were lower than the control group (Yen, 2009; Brevetti and Schiano, 2006).

The effects of different types of *Qi Gong* on diabetes patients have been studied. The Beijing Guang-on-mun Hospital, in collaboration with Japanese clinicians, conducted a clinical study on 108 type 2 diabetic patients, divided into four different groups: Group 1 practiced stretching *Qi Gong*; Group 2 practiced static *Qi Gong* (without stretching); Group 3 practiced both stretching and static *Qi Gong* and Group 4 was the control, not practicing *Qi Gong*. Observations lasted four months. Parameters included fasting blood sugar, and quality of Life (QoL) indices. Assessments were done before training, two and four months after training. The best results were observed in group 3 where all parameters, including objective blood tests and QoL improved after four months' training and the results were better than the control group. Results of the Group 1 and Group 3 also showed similar but less impressive trends (Lin and Wang, 2009).

In 2002, psychologists in Jiangxi conducted a research on the cognitive state and mental ability of elderly people aged 50–70, before and after six months' Qi Gong training. The assessment tool used was a software invented by Suen *et al.* in 1989, which tested the mental speed taken to solve simple mathematical problems, identification of symbols and sketches, motor reactions, memory, and imitations. It was shown that the hemoglobin A1c mental ability of the *Qi Gong* group improved significantly compared with the untrained group (Chang *et al.*, 2006; Suen *et al.*, 1989).

For all musculoskeletal training, motor improvement could mean positive effects on the bones as well. The Shantung Technical University has conducted a research on 60 people with known osteoporosis in 2008. The study group practiced *Qi Gong* daily for a period of 60 minutes, assessment included pain symptoms on an analog scale, bone mineral density measurement, serum alkaline phosphatase and other bone metabolism parameters. The end results after training (exact duration not given) showed significant improvement in bone health and bone mineral density.

11.7.2 *Tai Chi*

It might seem beyond any body's doubt that *Tai Chi* exercises will have general, as well as musculoskeletal effects on those who diligently practice it. The impression could be that it is particularly suitable for the elderly people. *Tai Chi* is certainly more popular than *Qi Gong*, although the three components: stretching, controlled breathing and meditation, are common to both. The dancing movements of *Tai Chi* could be the real motivating force for beginners.

Studies have shown that not only would disease-free people find benefits with the *Tai Chi* training, but those suffering from musculoskeletal weaknesses, e.g. after chronic work-related back injuries, could rely on *Tai Chi* exercises either as a solitary form of treatment, or as adjuvant therapy. One well-designed study was completed in two hospitals in Shanxi. 64 patients suffering from work-related spinal degeneration unrelated to other organic pathology were divided into two groups at random. One

Table 11.2. Treatment results in 4, 8, 12 weeks (Chen, 2009).

Group	Number	Male/Female	Recovered	Improved	No improvement	Cure rate	Effectiveness (%)
4 weeks							
Control	32	20/12	2	27	3	6.3	90.6
Tai Chi	32	22/10	4	28	1	9.4	96.9
8 weeks	32	20/12	40	21	1	31.3	96.9
Control	32	22/10	18	14	0	56.3[*a]	100
Tai Chi							
12 weeks							
Control	32	20/12	22	10	0	68.8	100
Tai Chi	32	22/10	27	5	0	84.4[*b]	100

[*a] $p < 0.01$; [*b] $p < 0.05$.

group was instructed to use *Tai Chi* as training, the other group received massage and physiotherapy. Results of treatment indicated positive benefits with *Tai Chi* at different stages of treatment (Chen, 2009; Shao and Zhou, 2008) (Table 11.2).

Tai Chi should be particularly good for training muscle balance in the lower limbs. A large scale comparative study was done in Beijing, covering 421 people on regular *Tai Chi* practice and others not doing sports. The study aimed at revealing whether *Tai Chi* would improve balancing power. A single test of one leg stand with blinded vision was used. The durations of stance was taken as objective data. Results showed uniform improvement in the *Tai Chi* group.

In this study, the method of assessing balance appeared too crude, and the differences between training and without training could be repeated using other assessment methodology (Taggart *et al.*, 2003; Maki, 1990).

Like *Qi Gong*, *Tai Chi* is known to have cardio-pulmonary supporting effects on the trainees. A study was conducted in Fujian on 39 middle aged and elderly people before and after they started training, which lasted one year. Using the cardiac function monitor, the following data were collected: stroke volume (SV), stroke index (SI), Cardiac output (CO), pulse rate (PR), heart oxygen consumption volume (HOV), and heart oxygen consumption index (HOI). The results are summarized in Table 11.3 (Lui *et al.*, 2001).

Table 11.3. Changes in cardiac function (Lui *et al.*, 2001).

Indice	1996	1997	Rate
PR (min)	76.18 ± 11.73	72.08 ± 9.18**	5.38
SV (ml)	81.14 ± 1.72	84.05 ± 16.86*	3.59
CO (L/min)	6.10 ± 1.05	6.42 ± 1.20*	5.29
SI (ml/m^2)	53.15 ± 9.51	55.41 ± 7.52*	4.24
HOI	2629.74 ± 616.08	2517.58 ± 593.45*	4.27
HOV (ml/min)	43.82 ± 10.27	40.23 ± 6.94*	8.19

*$p < 0.05$, **$p < 0.01$.

If *Tai Chi* is good for cardiac health, what about its effect on hypertension? The general mediating effects of exercises on hypertensive individuals are well accepted. Researchers from Sichuan have done a study on 124 patients suffering from essential hypertension, encouraging them to do *Tai Chi* exercises or therapeutic walking as means to help the standard drug treatment. Both groups showed positive effects with exercises, but the *Tai Chi* group did better. Patients with milder increases in blood pressure also did better than those with severe hypertension (Wang *et al.*, 2007; Mao, 2002; Werton, 2002; Wang, 2002).

Since *Tai Chi* helps with hypertension, one could assume that the complex system of stretching, controlled breathing and mediation, has humoral effects like controlling serum fatty acids and immunological influences. Public health experts in Sichuan University studied 72 Tai Chi exercisers and 55 controls to look at their serum antioxidants, *viz.* superoxide dismutase (SOD), glutathione peroxidase (GSH-Px), catalase (CAT) and malondialdehyde (MDA). Results showed that SOD, GSH-Px and CAT functions in the control group were higher than the *Tai Chi* group ($p < 0.05$) while MDA was lower ($p < 0.05$). Looking at the differences between the exercises of different durations, it is interesting to note that the longer the practice and experience, the more active were the antioxidants (Table 11.4) (Huang *et al.*, 2001; Tao and Tung, 1988).

Groups of gerontologist observed in recent years that deteriorating health and decline of physical performance of elderly people are often related to subclinical deficiencies of endocrine functions, particularly of the thyroid gland and gonads. Sports scientists in Shanghai investigated 51 elderly *Tai Chi* exercisers (60–90 years), comparing them with

Table 11.4. Relationship between different duration of *Tai Chi* practice (Huang *et al.*, 2001).

Markers	1–5 years		5–10 years		Over 10 years	
	n	$x \pm s$	n	$x \pm s$	n	$x \pm s$
SOD (NU/m l)	37	78.28 ± 15.27	21	99.66 ± 13.16	13	104.1 ± 12.48
GSH-Px (U/m l)	36	58.08 ± 2.88	22	72.21 ± 11.52	13	77.79 ± 8.75
CA T (U/m l)	37	1.78 ± 0.20	21	2.02 ± 0.19	13	2.05 ± 0.14
MDA (nmol/m l)	29	4.54 ± 0.19	10	4.03 ± 0.39	8	3.62 ± 0.17

Differences all reaching $p < 0.05$.

47 elderly (60–80 years) and 17 young adults (24–50 years). Serum markers included testosterone (T), estrogen (E2), luteohormone (LH), follicular stimulating hormone (FSH), thyroid stimulating hormone (TSH), thyroxin 4 (T4) and prolactin (PRL). Table 11.5 shows the interesting results, indicating decline in the hormone levels, with age. However, *Tai Chi* helps to alleviate some of the deficiencies (Hsu and Wang, 1986).

Like *Qi Gong*, *Tai Chi* is believed to have preventive function against infection and other pathological changes. Investigating immunology related changes should throw light on the assumption. The interleukins (IL's) are a group of cytokines created by mononuclear cells regulating cellular activities. IL2 is probably the most important member which controls the survival of T cells, NK cells and B cells, and is actively involved in anti-cancer activities.

Scholars in the College of Martial Arts, Beijing, have carried out a study to investigate the interleukin changes in 16 health women, aged between 55 and 65. Ten were *Tai Chi* exercisers while 6 were controls. After six months of exercises, the exercise group, which already had higher concentration of IL2, showed further increases. For those who already finished six months of *Tai Chi* training, even one single round of *Tai Chi* exercises, lasting one hour, boosted up the IL2 level to a statistically significant degree (from 100.3 ±20.46 to 110.7±20, p < 0.01) (Wang, 2003; Lewicki, 1988).

One of the intended effects of *Tai Chi* is a state of psychological balance like *Qi Gong*. Some studies have been designed to look at the contribution of *Tai Chi* on the psychological state of exercisers. 133 elderly people were recruited in Xian. They were divided into three groups of: *Tai Chi* practice, free exercisers, and control group with no exercises.

Table 11.5. Differences in serum hormone level (Hsu, 1986).

Serum Hormone Level	Tai Chi Group	Elderly Group	Young Group	p A:B	B:C	A:C
F (ng/dl)	14.74 ± 4.73	15.23 ± 7.67	14.20 ± 3.92	> 0.05	> 0.05	> 0.05
TSH (μU/ml)	4.80 ± 3.05	3.80 ± 1.55	3.10 ± 1.15	< 0.05	> 0.05	< 0.05
T_3 (ng/ml)	0.93 ± 0.20	0.84 ± 0.21	1.51 ± 0.31	< 0.05	< 0.01	< 0.05
T_4 (ng/ml)	69.97 ± 23.87	73.60 ± 31.96	104.97 ± 38.60	> 0.05	< 0.05	< 0.01
rT_3 (ng/ml)	30.26 ± 7.77	28.79 ± 4.96	37.22 ± 7.64	> 0.05	< 0.01	< 0.01
FSH (mIU/ml)	16.54 ± 15.16	11.05 ± 6.08	4.85 ± 1.58	< 0.05	< 0.01	< 0.01
LH (mIU/ml)	11.74 ± 13.19	8.03 ± 5.95	4.41 ± 1.31	> 0.05	< 0.01	< 0.05
T (ng/dl)	$680.00 \pm 430.00^*$	510.00 ± 151.00	$679.00 \pm 173.00^{**}$	< 0.05	< 0.01	> 0.05
E_2 (pg/ml)	63.91 ± 17.14	$54.74 \pm 18.62^{\Delta}$	$50.70 \pm 7.14^{\Delta\Delta}$	< 0.05	> 0.05	< 0.05
PRL (ng/ml)	7.06 ± 3.46	6.34 ± 2.75	8.25 ± 3.21	> 0.05	> 0.05	> 0.05

* $n = 50$; ** $n = 12$; $^{\Delta}$ $n = 46$; $^{\Delta\Delta}$ $n = 10$.

Their psychological states were assessed at zero, two, and six months, using the Cornell University Mental Assessment index (CMA). With this assessment index, psychological explorations included symptoms of depression, anxiety and tension. Included in the questionnaire were also symptoms of the vital systems: respiratory, cardiovascular, gastro-intestinal, muscular-skeletal, neurological, etc. Frequency of fatigue and illnesses was also explored. The results of the study showed a general improvement on the psychological parameters, reaching statistical significance, while the other functional indices are also shown to the advantage of the *Tai Chi* group (Yi, 2008).

11.8 Conclusions

We have briefly reviewed the history of Natural Healing in China, its philosophical background, conceptualization within the practice of Chinese Medicine, the procedural requirements, claims and recent scientific endeavours to reveal the physiological basis of the two most popular exercises, *viz. Qi Gong* and *Tai Chi*. It would be appropriate to give more general discussions, and to approach more from the common sense aspect so as to try answering one question — "Should I practice *Qi Gong* or *Tai Chi*?"

Natural Healing in Europe and US might have specific demands and needs. Natural Healing in the oriental sense is more of a promotion of wellness and longevity, although those people threatened by diseases or ill-health might have their special needs and demands. We might not feel particularly threatened by the imagination of a special disease, but we certainly do not want to fall sick. We might not particularly adore and work for longevity, but again, we do not want to fall sick. If not falling sick could be achieved through the simple procedures of stretching exercises, controlled breathing and meditation, it would certainly be most inviting. If the tripartite procedures can be easily learned, comfortably practiced and more importantly, freely modified, they would earn even greater popularity and deserve more promotions.

Looking at the modifications of the procedures involved in the exercises throughout the long period of its history, we could be quite confident about the flexibility that could be allowed. Since stretching exercises with different postures have been practiced and recorded over 3000 years ago, countless numbers of practice system have evolved, bearing the same principles. All those systems of exercises, labelled with unique names of their own, have enjoyed genuine popularities and substantial groups of followers. When instructors take up the role of training new students, they naturally have a tendency to modify again the details. Afterall, not a single individual could claim the ability to exactly perform a muscular (motor) action that exactly matched another person's performance. Modification and diversion is therefore mandatory. After so many decades of intentional and unintentional modifications, exercises like *Qi Gong* and *Tai Chi* have retained their Natural Healing values. Individual modifications, as long as they are conforming to the basic concepts and requirements, should be allowed, even encouraged. Although different groups have rather rigid directions and contents of training and followers are instructed to closely follow, when they fail to do so perfectly, they are allowed to modify along their own abilities. If the system of exercises could be so freely modified, does it mean that individuals could just be acquainted with the procedures, adhere to the basic principles, and then creatively practice on their own?

I realize that different groups in China, on their own pursue of Natural Healing, have already done that. The evidence could be found in the public parks in China today. Early in the morning in these parks, one finds people practicing conventional *Qi Gong* and *Tai Chi*. One finds also other groups practicing other innovative forms of stretching exercises which they have invented. One sees them engaged in modified folk dancing, social dancing, different stretches, etc. There are also those who walk with their backs leading the way. These are all innovative inventions of exercises basing on the principle of stretching.

What about the other area of controlled breathing? There are groups of people practicing singing, or Peking opera. Others shout and/or yell in their own way of control, making colourful innovative varieties of controlled breathing. A few quietly Buddha-sit below the trees and are engaged in either conventional or their own way of controlled respiration. *Qi Gong* instructions have listed a variety of breathing patterns with short or long lengths at different stages of the breathing cycle and to be performed with different forces, through the chest cage or abdominal diaphragm. The varieties of advocated breathing patterns, in fact, have indirectly endorsed the feasibility of individualized innovative practices and have apparently encouraged the practices of singing and yelling.

Our current attitude could be: the practice of stretching and controlled breathing, after all, promotes physical and psychological well-being that aspires to a superb tranquility of the mind, could be recommended to all. In fact it could be a happy coincidence that the same requirements, *viz.* stretching, controlled breathing and meditation, are required in the popular Health Promotion exercise in India: the Yoga practice.

While the practice of Natural Healing in the Chinese Community is historical and cultural, it is also very personal. It is a personal habit that the individual has chosen to adopt. In a way it resembles eating habit and sleeping habit that do not need any justification. Still, the individual could review it with the intension of modification or enforcement for one's own good. Scientific proof for the practice of *Qi Gong* and *Tai Chi* on one's well-being would not be required. However, nowadays, even well-being — wellness, could be physiologically or clinically defined and objective parameters are created for the measurement of wellness. Those who are converted to thorough, strict scientific explorations have started investigating the "objective value" of *Qi Gong*, *Tai Chi* and other Natural Healing practices.

I have already given examples of proper research studies reported from different institutions in China. From those reports, scattered evidences of favourable changes in various physiological areas have been shown. In fact, the interest on the Chinese way of Natural Healing has turned international. Japanese scholars have reported widely on the cardio pulmonary effects of *Qi Gong* and *Tai Chi*, as well as their immuno-modulating influences (Li and Chu, 2008; Chen and Chang, 2002). Likewise, the most influential research institution on health, NIH, USA, has many times encouraged research commitment on *Qi Gong* and *Tai Chi*. A recent report from NIH about a randomized controlled trial of 112 subjects aged 59–86 on *Tai Chi* exercises, against health education, using chicken pox vaccine as a stimulant to immunological responses, indicated that the *Tai Chi* group enjoyed a 40% increase in their immunological responses (double to that of the controls), and an improved physical and mental state of health (Irwin and Olmstead, 2007).

Let us go back to the basic question of "Should I practice *Qi Gong* or *Tai Chi?*"

The popularity is clear. The popularity is historically and culturally linked. The practice requires little cost. The practice can be easily verified at different levels of personal practice.

But if one considers that scientific proof is of paramount importance, what we are clear today, remains scanty, non-specific, and partial.

May be there is a hidden concept that could be revealed through careful observations on the practice of *Qi Gong* and *Tai Chi*: particularly its procedures of stretching, controlled breathing and meditation.

What does stretching do? Stretching produces tension on the muscles, tendons, ligaments and the components of the joints. Stretching with chosen positions produces tension on some muscles, tendons, ligaments and joints that are normally not for active use. The Gate Theory in neurophysiology confers that with every stretch and stimulation of the proprioceptive nerve receptor in the tendons and ligaments, messages are sent up to the brain to block up pain sensation and initiate other chains of events in the central nervous system. With every intensional stretch additional proprioceptive messages are sent up. When people walk backwards with their backs leading the way, what are happening? Muscle groups that are not normally active in walking are activated and they send out massive unusual proprioceptive messages to the brain.

What does controlled breathing do? Controlled breathing creates an unusual motor system for respiratory function which follows a new sequence and pattern. The modified rates, intensities of inspiration and expiration, the different groups of muscles mobilized, together composed a totally novel, inexperienced system of motor activity. Stimulations received through these complex motor activities are new to the central nervous system. The stimulation is not only confined to the accustomed somatosensory system of neurological control. The respiratory control is mastered through both the somatic motor system, which allows voluntary control, and the autonomic (parasympathetic) nervous system, which is responsible for the automatic regulatory control of respiration. Intentional controlled breathing therefore is making use of the somatic nervous activity to initiate stimulation on the autonomic nervous system, which has wide connections with the internal organs. Controlled breathing therefore opens up new channels of communication with the internal organs under rational intension. These new channels of communication, could give an explanation to the old concept of *Qi Gong* and *Tai Chi*, that the practice pushes the *qi* through the internal organs to help building a state of physiological harmony.

What does meditation do? No one is free from the somatic stimulations and psychological disturbances that bother him endlessly. One does enjoy a good rest during night time sleep. Unfortunately, with overloads of accumulative worldly events, even night rests are frequently challenged. Achieving extra moments of spiritual tranquility is a blessing for all. Buddhists, monks and priests have means and experience acquiring the spiritual tranquility. *Qi Gong* and *Tai Chi* practices aim at the same achievement. Through the practice of stretching and controlled breathing, that state of mind is expected to automatically come. Is this a myth? Should one need to reach the mental state of a fervent religious follower before one reaches such a spiritual state? May be the extraordinary neurological inputs from stretching and controlled respiration are the hidden benefactors pushing toward the state of tranquility. Firstly, stretching controls any pain (through the Gate theory), eliminates stiffness, relaxes the musculoskeletal components, thus removes adverse somatic inputs and initiates pleasant humoral exchanges within the brain. Secondly, the controlled breathing mobilizes independent autonomic nervous pathways which help to adjust contradicting physiological activities at humoral levels. The outcome of the unusual input from the two normally uncoordinated systems of neurological activities could be a novel state of harmony between the body and mind.

With this obviously optimistic, yet over-simplified concept in mind, one could confidently start ones own personal practice of Natural Healing, using any form of *Qi Gong* or *Tai Chi*. One may even invent his own practice as long as the activities consist of stretching, controlled breathing and meditation.

How is Qi Gong and Tai Chi different from aerobic exercises? Aerobic exercises aim at the training of skeletal muscles which directly pull on the joints in the normal day to day fashion. As much energy is needed, oxygen consumption needs to be sharply increased. The result is a need for a parallel increase in the efficacy of the lungs and the heart. The rationale of aerobic exercises, therefore, is to engage in a comprehensive training of musculo - skeleto - cardio - pulmonary function (Whelton, 2002). All those are normal day-to-day physiological functions. In contrast, *Qi Gong* and *Tai Chi* consist of static exercises coupled with a variable amount of dynamic moves. A lot of unusual, extraordinary neurological stimulations are elicited through the stretching and stimulation of muscles and ligaments. The controlled respirations elicit autonomic nervous stimulations which again, do not happen normally. Henceforth, the mental state of tranquility obtained through *Qi Gong* and *Tai Chi* is something unimaginable for anyone doing strenuous aerobic exercises.

Aerobic exercises have limitations, not only during performance, but also in the long term. Over strenuous musculoskeletal training is going to damage the joints. In fact, biomechanical studies have indicated that if jogging exceeds the frequency of one mile per day and three times per week, cartilage damages will be inevitable. In the case of *Qi Gong* and *Tai Chi*, limitations on the physiological ability during the training are virtually unknown, and in the long term, the joints involved do not suffer any threatening damages.

What about other means advocated for the practice of Natural Healing like special food and botanicals?

It is true that Natural Healing involves food and botanicals in both European and Chinese Practices. Food and botanicals are considered "natural" because they occur in Nature in spite of the fact that feeding individuals with special purposes does not appear that "natural". When the oldest Chinese Medicine classic *Ne-jing* discussed Natural Healing: only stretching, controlled breathing and meditation are emphasized again and again. Use of other means like botanicals, are additional measures created by subsequent clinicians when either exercises fails to give the desirable effects or more rapid responses are needed for various reasons.

Qi Gong, and *Tai Chi* could therefore be taken as the essential practices leading to Natural Healing and Longevity while botanicals can be used as supportive, secondary tools.

References

Astsumi, K. (2007) Integrative approach towards "healthy aging". In: *Proceedings of "Inter Natural Symposium on Healthy Aging"*. Tokyo University Press, Tokyo, pp. 2–5.

Brevetti, G. and Schiano, V. (2006) Cellular adhesion molecules and peripheral arterial disease. *Vasc. Med.* **11**(1), 39–47.

Chang, C. and Wai, S. (1997) Tai Chi and physiology of middle and old aged people. *J. Binzhou Med. Coll.* **20**(5), 505.

Chang, W.C., Zhung, T.B. and Wu, C.H. (2006) Qi gong and cognitive changes. *Chin. J. Behav. Med. Sci.* **15**(9), 827–828.

Chen, J.H. (1998) Natural healing and *tai chi*. *World Sci. Tech.* **5**, 15–18.

Chen, M.K. (2009) Qi gong and osteoporosis. *Consuma Guide Tech. Forum* **10**, 217–218.

Chen, W.Z. and Chang, T. (2002) *Qi gong* and hand temperature. *J. Int. Soc. Life Inform. Sci.* **20**(2), 707–110.

Du, S.W., Chang, C.L. and Wang, S. (2006) Qi gong and cardiac function of middle and old age people. *Chin J. Sports Med.* **25**(6), 721–726.

Green, D.J. and Blankshy, B.A. (1996) Control skeletal muscle blood flow during dynamic exercise. *J. Sports Med.* **21**, 119–146.

Hsu, H.F. (1986) Qi Gong and immunological indices. *Qi Gong* **6**, 279–283.

Hsu, S.W. and Wang, W.J. (1986) Tai chi and internal secretion. *China J. Phys. Med.* **5**(3), 150–153.

Huang, J. (2009) History, current situation and future of stretching exercises in disease prevention. *J. Beijing Univ. Tradit. Chin. Med.* **32**(9), 586–589.

Huang, Y.H., Leong, Y.F. and Jim, C.L. (2001) *Tai chi* influence on elderly people's serum anti oxidants. *Occup. Health Inj.* **16**(3), 139–141.

Irwin, M.R. and Olmstead, R. (2007) Augmenting immune responses to varicella zoster virus in older adults: A randomized controlled trial of *tai chi*. *J. Am. Geriatr. Soc.* **55**, 511–517.

Ji, L.Z. (1994a) Natural healing in Chinese medicine. *Beijing Chin. Med. J.* **1**, 62–63.

Ji, L.Z. (1994b) Natural healing in Chinese medicine. *Beijing Chin. Med. J.* **2**, 62–63.

Ji, L.Z. (1994c) Natural healing in Chinese medicine. *Beijing Chin. Med. J.* **3**, 61–63.

Ji, L.Z. (1994d) Natural healing in Chinese medicine. *Beijing Chin. Med. J.* **4**, 63–65.

Ji, L.Z. (1994e) Natural healing in Chinese medicine. *Beijing Chin. Med. J.* **5**, 63–64.

Jones, B.M. (2001) Change in cytokine production in healthy subjects practicing *qi gong*: A pilot study. *J. Complement. Altern. Med.* **1**, 8–10.

Lewicki, E. (1988) Effects of maximal physical exercise on T lymphocyte subpopulations and on interleukin 1 (IL 1) and interleukin 2 (IL 2) production *in vitro*. *Int. J. Sports Med.* **9**(2), 114–117.

Li, S.C. and Chu, W.C. (2008) Recent scientific research on *qi gong* in Japan. *Rep. Relat. Chin. Med. Outside China* **25**(5), 276–279.

Liang, X.S. (2005) Natural healing. *J. Xiaolin Tai Chi* **1**, 53.

Lic, S. (2003) Four ways of natural healing I and II. *Natural Healing Monthly* (養生月刊) Feb. & Mar.

Lin, W.N. and Wang, W.T. (2009) Natural healing and type 2 diabetes. *Beijing J. Tradit. Chin. Med.* **28**(1), 9–12.

Lui, S.S., Yi, H.A. and Chen, C.Y. (2001) Tai chi and cardio pulmonary function. *Modern Rehabil.* **5**(6) 64–65.

Maki, B.E. (1990) Aging and postural control. *J. Am. Geriatr. Soc.* **38**(1), 1–9.

Mao, C. (2002) Influence of exercise training on elderly people with borderline hypertension. *Chin. J. Clin. Rehabil.* **6**(11), 1673–1676.

Motoyama, M. and Sunami, Y. (1998) Low intensity aerobic training in elderly hypertensive people. *J. Med. Sci. Sport Exerc.* **30**(6), 818–813.

Shao, L. and Zhou, Y. (2008) Tai chi and work injury back pain. *J. Shanxi Normal Univ.* **36**(5), 35–36.

Si, H.Y. (2006) Fitness qi gong of health. *Chin. J. Clin. Rehabil.* **10**(47), 145–147.

Suen, L.F., Lui, S.P. and Hsu, J.H. (1989) Clinical evaluation of declining cognitive power — Application in research of TCM. *J. Integr. Med.* **9**, 203–207.

Taggart, H.M., Arslanian, C.L., Bae, S. and Singh, K. (2003) Effects of Tai Chi exercise on fibromyalgia symptoms and health-related quality of life. *Orthop. Nurs.* **22**(5), 353–360.

Tao, G.S. and Tung, W. (1988) Indices of aging. *China J. Geriatr. Med.* **7**(3), 167–172.

Tsang, Y.K. and Chow, S.C. (2005) Natural healing and physiological changes of middle and elderly age people. *J. Beijing Sport Univ.* **28**(9), 1206–1209.

Wang, K.H. (2008) Historical changes of natural healing exercises in China. *Sports Culture J.* **3** (體育文化專刊).

Wang, C. (2007) Natural healing in Chinese medicine. *Scholast. Rev.* (學習時報) **7**, 23–25.

Wang, C.J. (2003) Tai chi and interleukins. *J. Shantung Inst. Sport* **19**(2), 48–30.

Wang, L. and Xiang, L.J. (2006) Principles of Chinese medicine and *tai chi*. *J. Shanxi Coll. Tradit. Chin. Med.* **29**(5), 4–6.

Wang, T., Lu, W. and Wu, Z.Y. (2007) Hypertension rehabilitated with walking or *tai chi*. *Modern Prevent. Med.* **34**(18), 3535–3543.

Wang, Y. (2002) *Tai chi* and hypertension of the elderly. *J. Marshal Art Sci.* **1**(4), 47–52.

Whelton, S.P. (2002) Effects of aerobic exercise on blood pressure: A meta-analysis of randomized controlled trials. *Ann. Int. Med.* **136**, 493–503.

Won, J.C. (2004) Natural healing and *tai chi*. *Anhui J. Sport Tech.* **9**, 93–95.

Won, X.S. (2008) Natural healing review. *Tai Chi Rev.* **11**, 29–30.

Yang, W. (2001) Natural healing and *tai chi*. *J. Fujian Coll. Tradit. Chin. Med.* **2**, 56–57.

Yen, Y. (2009) Qi gong influence on serum fatty acids. *J. Liaoning Normal Univ.* **32**(3), 356–358.

Yi, L.O. (2008) *Tai chi* and elderly health. *China J. Health Psychol.* **16**(4), 477–478.

Yi, X.K. (2007) Natural healing in Chinese medicine. *World Health Digest* **4**, 269–270.

Chapter 12

The Status of Yoga Research in India

Shirley Telles and Naveen K. Visweswaraiah

Abstract

Yoga is an ancient Indian way of life which includes specific practices, postures, voluntarily regulated breathing, meditation and philosophical principles. In India research on the effects of yoga began in the 1920s and continues today. While studies on the physiological effects of different practices are the most numerous (but have not been described here as they do not have direct applications), there is also research on the applications of yoga. The most common application is as a form of add-on therapy for a wide range of disorders. These studies have attempted to assess whether yoga is useful or not, and in some cases possible mechanisms have also been studied. Other applications (for example in adaptation to unusually stressful environments) and the use of yoga for stress management are also mentioned. This review has attempted to cover a wide range of applications of yoga practice in different parts of the country. Though there is a possibility that some studies may have been omitted the review shows that the applications of yoga in health are many and varied and are being actively explored.

Keywords: Yoga; Regulated Breathing; Meditation; Stress Relief; Therapy; Environmental Adaptions.

12.1 Early Studies Investigating Special Powers in Accomplished Practitioners

The earliest research in yoga began in the 1920s. Experiments were conducted by Swami Kuvalayananda and the observations were meticulously noted in a journal (*Yoga Mimamsa*) (Kuvalayananda, 1925). What was particularly interesting was that these studies examined fairly complex yoga techniques (e.g., two techniques which involve contraction of the abdominal muscles *nauli* and *agnisara*), and used assessment techniques which were relatively novel at the time, such as X-rays and measurements of the barometric pressure within the viscera. This period of meticulous research was followed by research on the special powers which yogis attain after dedicated and committed practice, which are called *siddhis*. Examples of *siddhis* include being able to remain without oxygen for surprisingly long periods or being able to stop the heart beating at will. While there were several studies on practitioners with these supposed powers, very few studies actually supported the claims. These have been described below.

At the All India Institute of Medical Sciences (A.I.I.M.S.), New Delhi, India, Anand, Chhina and Singh (1961) recorded the changes when a yogi was confined in an airtight box. Recordings were made twice. First, a burning candle was placed inside the box and the yogi remained in the box for eight hours. Second, the yogi remained in the box for ten hours without the burning candle. On both occasions he did not develop tachycardia or hyperpnea. In the same year, a study was conducted to compare the ability to voluntarily control the heart beat through yoga, with the control being the Valsalva maneuver (Wenger, Bagchi, and Anand, 1961). In one out of four yogis the heart rate slowed down. Based on this the authors assumed that as a result of some voluntary muscular mechanism, vagal input to the sino-atrial node had interrupted the regular cardiac cycles.

12.2   A Novel Approach: Studies on Less Experienced and Naïve-to-Yoga Persons

The idea of confining yoga research to experienced yogis with special attainments was radically altered when a sage from India, Maharishi Mahesh Yogi introduced Transcendental Meditation (TM) to the world (Maharishi Mahesh Yogi, 1966). The effects of practicing this relatively simple technique in people who had no previous experience of meditation led to a shift in the focus of yoga research (Wallace, 1970).

In the early 1980s, another important step in yoga research was taken by the Indian Council of Medical Research (the apex body for medical research in India), which funded a multi-faceted project to understand the neurophysiological changes in *pranayamas* and meditations at the National Institute of Mental Health and Neurosciences (NIMHANS, in Bangalore in south India) (Desiraju, 1983). The assessment methods used were, at the time, state-of-the-art assessment techniques, including different modalities of evoked potentials, fast-Fourier transform analysis of the electroencephalogram [EEG], polysomnography, and various methods to assess neurotransmitter levels and their metabolites. The main research methodology innovation was that subjects were studied in repeat sessions to assess intra-individual variability and each subject was assessed in 'experimental' and 'control' sessions, rather than a comparison between yoga practitioners and a matched group of non-practitioners (i.e., a self-as-control design, rather than a matched groups design, which was used in most studies before this) (Telles, and Desiraju, 1993; Telles, Joseph, Venkatesh, and Desiraju, 1993).

12.3 Therapeutic Applications of Yoga

At approximately the same time there was a strong interest in the therapeutic applications of yoga. A cardiologist of Indian origin (Chandra Patel) carried out a series of rigorous, randomized controlled trials, which showed the usefulness of yoga as an add-on treatment in the management of hypertension when compared to conventional treatment and to biofeedback (Patel, 1975; Patel, and North, 1975). There was also an interest in other conditions, considered to be psychosomatic in origin. For example, a randomized controlled trial showed that a combination of yoga practices (including yoga postures, voluntary regulated breathing [*pranayama*], meditation, and certain philosophical principles) was beneficial in bronchial asthma (Nagarathna, and Nagendra, 1985). Other studies examined whether specific practices used individually would have a beneficial effect. For example, a cleansing technique (called *kunjal*) which involves induced emesis, reduced nocturnal symptoms in bronchial asthmatics during the week the practice was performed (Singh, 1987). The same author also examined the effect of voluntary regulated yoga breathing in persons with mild bronchial asthma (Singh *et al.*, 1990). This study was the first and remains the only placebo-controlled study in yoga research, as a placebo for yoga practice is difficult to devise. In this study, participants were asked to breathe through an active device (which made the device resemble *pranayama* by regulating the inhalation: exhalation ratio as 1:2), while the other group breathed through a 'passive' device, which had no effect on breathing. The group who breathed through the 'active' device showed a significantly lower response (i.e., bronchoconstriction) to histamine.

Indians are considered particularly susceptible to hypertension and coronary heart disease. An early study showed that relaxation while supine in the corpse posture (*shavasana*) was effective in the management of hypertension (Datey *et al.*, 1969). There was a major shift in thinking about the management of coronary artery disease, following the epoch-making study of Dean Ornish from the University of California, San Fransisco, which showed that a change in lifestyle can effectively reverse coronary artery disease (Ornish, 1983). Subsequently and more recently there have been two studies from separate groups in India which showed that yoga-based lifestyle changes can help in the retardation of coronary atherosclerosis (Manchanda *et al.*, 2000), as well as in the reversal of ischemic heart disease (Yogendra *et al.*, 2004). In the first study (Manchanda *et al.*, 2000), 42 men angiographically proven to have coronary artery disease were randomized as a control ($n = 21$) and a yoga intervention group ($n = 21$), with a follow-up after a year. The intervention consisted of yoga, control of risk factors, diet control, and moderate aerobic exercise. The control group was managed by conventional methods (i.e., risk factor control and prescribed diet changes). At the end of a year the yoga group showed a significant reduction in number of angina episodes per week, improved exercise capacity and decrease in body weight. Serum total cholesterol, LDL cholesterol and triglyceride levels reduced to a greater degree in the yoga group who also required revascularization procedures (i.e., coronary angioplasty or bypass surgery) less frequently. Also, coronary angiography repeated at one year showed that more lesions regressed and fewer lesions progressed in the yoga group. In the subsequent study (Yogendra *et al.*, 2004), 113 angiographically proven coronary artery disease patients were assessed at the beginning and end of a year during which the yoga group ($n = 71$) had a program which included control of risk factors, dietary modifications and stress management. This resulted in a significant reduction in total cholesterol, LDL cholesterol, and regression of the disease and arrest of progression.

Another condition to which Indians are considered particularly susceptible is diabetes mellitus. As for coronary artery disease (described above), yoga-based lifestyle modifications, have been showed useful in the management of diabetes (Sahay, and Sahay, 2002; Sahay, 2007).

Possible mechanisms by which yoga may be of benefit in diabetes include increasing insulin sensitivity (Chaya *et al.*, 2008). Another possible mechanism is by modulating leptin sensitivity (Telles *et al.*, 2010).

Another area which has been of interest in India is whether yoga can help in alcoholism, which is a cause of loss of productivity and morbidity, and is especially damaging to those belonging to low income groups. An early study found that yoga, including meditation, was one among different novel methods of treatment (e.g., non-volitional biofeedback) found to be useful in managing alcoholism with a one year follow-up period (Subramanyam *et al.*, 1986).

Subsequently, a yoga program which consisted of rhythmic yoga breathing, called *Sudarshan Kriya Yoga* (SKY) was found useful (Vedamurthachar *et al.*, 2006). Following a week of conventional detoxification management strategies consenting subjects were randomized as a SKY group and a control group. After two weeks of intervention the SKY group showed a greater decrease in depression, and changes in plasma cortisol and ACTH suggestive of a shift towards normalcy.

Another study conducted in a residential setting assessed the effect of ninety days of *Kundalini yoga* program on persons with a history of substance abuse (Khalsa *et al.*, 2008). Subjects showed improvements on a several psychological self-report questionnaires.

While the benefits of yoga for alcoholism have been described above, yoga practice has also been investigated for other psychological disorders. These include depression, anxiety (as well as neuroticism) and post-traumatic stress disorder [PTSD].

The rhythmic yoga breathing (called *Sudarshan Kriya Yoga* or SKY mentioned above) was shown to as useful as tricyclic antidepressants (e.g., imipramine) in managing depression, though it was found inferior to electro-convulsive therapy (Janakiramaiah *et al.*, 2009).

In addition to yoga breathing techniques, a meditation technique called *Sahaj Yoga* was found beneficial in patients with major depression when practiced for eight weeks (Sharma *et al.*, 2005). It was also seen that when the practice of *Sahaj Yoga* was added to conventional antidepressant medication, patients with major depression showed improvement in executive functions like processing of information related to verbal working memory, improved attention span, and better visuo-motor speed (Sharma *et al.*, 2006). Apart from yoga breathing and meditation techniques considered individually, a combination of yoga practices were found useful to lower levels of depression in community dwelling older persons (Krishnamurthy and Telles, 2007). Finally, a randomized controlled trial was conducted which showed that over a four month period, diagnosed schizophrenics on anti-psychotic treatment showed less psychopathology when they practiced a combination of yoga practices compared to a group given physiotherapy, where both were add-on treatments (Duraiswami *et al.*, 2007). Anxiety, particularly state anxiety at the moment of testing was found to decrease in persons seeking stress relief with sessions of both yoga theory and yoga practice (Telles *et al.*, 2009).

Apart from this one week of yoga practice reduced symptoms of neuroticism in persons who had joined a yoga program for stress relief (Telles *et al.*, 2010). Finally in discussing yoga and mental health, there have been studies which have shown that yoga practice is useful in the management of post-traumatic stress disorder. Reduced fear, anxiety, disturbed sleep, and sadness were observed in survivors of the 2004 tsunami after they practiced yoga for one week (Telles *et al.*, 2007). Apart from this, a randomized controlled trial showed that a yoga breath intervention reduced symptoms related to trauma exposure also in tsunami survivors after six weeks of practice (Descilo *et al.*, 2009).

Even today, among various ailments and despite advancements in treatment, cancer is considered difficult to manage. Yoga practice has been shown to have a number of beneficial effects in oncology. The side effects of conventional treatment for cancer include chemotherapy-induced nausea and vomiting. Following yoga practiced as 60 minutes daily throughout chemotherapy, breast cancer patients had lower scores on a conventional scale for nausea and emesis, as well as less anxiety, depression and distress, compared to a control group who received supportive therapy (Raghavendra *et al.*, 2007). The same yoga practices modulated psychological stress and reduced radiation-induced genotoxic stress, also in breast cancer patients (Bannerjee *et al.*, 2007). An even earlier study showed that rhythmic yoga breathing alone, practiced for 24 weeks increased NK cell activity in cancer patients who had completed their standard treatment (Kochupillai *et al.*, 2005). This finding was supported by a later study (Rao *et al.*, 2008).

Yoga practice had also been shown to modify autonomic imbalances known to exist in epileptics, with a shift towards parasympathetic dominance and a decrease in seizure scores (Sathyaprabha *et al.*, 2008).

While we discussed stress-related diseases, cancer and psychiatric conditions all having a strong component of stress, a prospective, randomized trial (Visweswaraiah and Telles, 2004) explored the usefulness of yoga in an infectious disease which is a major burden in Asian countries i.e., pulmonary tuberculosis. This study compared the efficacy of anti-tuberculosis treatment (ATT) with two separate programs (yoga and breath awareness), on lung capacities and bacteriological status. In addition to ATT, one group practised yoga ($n = 25$) and the other practised breath awareness ($n = 23$) for six hours per week, each session being 60 minutes. At the end of two months, the yoga group showed a significant reduction in symptom scores (88.1%), an increase in weight (10.9%), FVC (64.7%) and FEV(1) (83.6%). The breath awareness group also showed a significant reduction in symptom scores (16.3%), and an increase in weight (2.1%) and FEV(1) (63.8%). Significantly more patients in the yoga group showed sputum conversion based on microscopy on days 30 and 45 compared to the breath awareness group. Ten of 13 in the yoga group had negative sputum culture after 60 days compared with four of 19 in the breath awareness group. Improvement in the radiographic picture occurred in 16/25 in the yoga group compared to 3/22 in the breath awareness group on day 60.

Hence the improved level of infection, radiographic picture, FVC, weight gain and reduced symptoms in the yoga group suggest a complementary role for yoga in the management of pulmonary tuberculosis.

12.4 Applications of Yoga in Physiological and Premorbid Conditions

The descriptions above have detailed some of the therapeutic applications of yoga for a wide range of disorders. A combination of yoga practices (the sun salutation [*suryanamaskar*], regulated breathing [*pranayama*] and meditation) decreased climacteric symptoms, perceived stress and neuroticism in perimenopausal women, when practiced for eight weeks (one hour daily, five days a week), compared to an equal duration of simple physical exercises (Chattha *et al.*, 2008).

Apart from menopause, which is a physiological condition, obesity which is now known to be a premorbid condition for different diseases, also responds favorably to yoga. Following a one week yoga and diet change program, obese persons showed a decrease in body mass index, waist and hip circumferences, total cholesterol, as well as reduced serum leptin and increased postural stability and grip strength (Telles *et al.*, 2010), There was, however, a decrease in HDL levels and in fat-free mass which were believed to be due to the sudden change to a plant-based diet, low in fat, as yoga practice (in studies done elsewhere) has been shown to increase HDL levels and fat-free mass.

12.4.1 *Effect of yoga on aging*

A three-arm randomized controlled trial was conducted on 69 community dwelling adults aged 60 years and above who had no physical or mental disorder. Several variables were assessed in them after they were randomized as a yoga group, an ayurveda group and a waitlist control group. There were a number of benefits seen in the yoga group, and some benefits in the ayurveda group (who received a polyherbal preparation twice a day).

One of the benefits seen was in the self-rated quality of sleep (Manjunath, and Telles, 2005). The yoga group showed a significant decrease in the time taken to fall asleep (approximate group average decrease was ten minutes), an increase in the total number of hours slept and in the feeling of being rested in the morning, based on a rating scale, after six months. The yoga group also showed a significant decrease in depression scores that were abnormally high at baseline after both three and six months of practice (Krishnamurthy and Telles, 2007a).

Another benefit seen by practicing yoga was an improvement in gait and balance based on the scores obtained from standard scales (Krishnamurthy and Telles, 2007b). More indirectly, both yoga and ayurveda appeared to have a protective effect on lung functions, as the control group showed a decrease in vital capacity after six months while the yoga and ayurveda groups did not (Manjunath and Telles, 2006).

Apart from this randomized controlled trial, a separate study examined the use of yoga along with other changes in lifestyle in the elderly (Arya, 2000). Also, a specific meditation technique (i.e., Brahmakumaris Raja Yoga Meditation) was shown to modify the lipid profile, hence lowering the risk of coronary artery disease in post-menopausal women (Vyas *et al.*, 2008).

12.4.2 *Yoga for stress management in students and specific occupations*

A study conducted on medical students showed that yoga practice reduces examination stress (Malathi and Damodaran, 1999). Among various occupations, professionals associated with information technology (IT) are considered vulnerable to specific stresses. These include mental stress, visual strain and musculoskeletal discomfort. Following two months of yoga (45 minutes daily, five days a week) professional computer users showed reduced visual strain (Telles *et al.*, 2006) as well as a lesser likelihood of developing somatic symptoms as a consequence of mental strain (Telles and Naveen, 2006).

12.4.3 *Other applications of yoga*

The northern boundary of India lies in inhospitable terrain and at high altitude. There are several army bases in this region and hence there has been an interest to determine whether practicing yoga can facilitate adapting to a high altitude with less discomfort and in a shorter time (Rawal *et al.*, 1994; Selvamurthy *et al.*, 1988).

Hence many and varied applications of yoga practice have been researched in India. The most important among these is the promotion of positive health. These have not been detailed here as the studies on the physiological effects of yoga in normal individuals are too numerous. However studies on the effects of yoga in the treatment of disease have been described.

It is encouraging to note that research on yoga which began almost a century ago in India, and continues to be of great interest in yoga institutions as well as in medical institutions of national importance. Equally encouraging is the fact that research in the area is being actively funded by the Government of India. It is important and fitting that research on the effects and applications of yoga is carried out with a maximum blend of knowledge of the traditional texts along with present-day scientific method.

Acknowledgments

The authors gratefully acknowledge the help of Mr. Nilkamal Singh and Mr. Sachin Sharma in preparing the manuscript.

References

Anand, B.K., Chhina, G.S. and Singh, B. (1961) Studies on Shri Ramanand Yogi during his stay in an air-tight box. *Indian J. Med. Res.* **49**, 82–89.

Arya, S.N. (2000) The problem of hypertension in the elderly. *J. Indian Med. Assoc.* **98**, 176–179.

Banerjee, B., Vadiraj, H.S., Ram, A., Rao, R., Jayapal, M., Gopinath, K.S., Ramesh, B.S., Rao, N., Kumar, A., Raghuram, N., Hegde, S., Nagendra, H.R. and Prakash Hande, M. (2007) Effects of an integrated yoga program in modulating psychological stress and radiation-induced genotoxic stress in breast cancer patients undergoing radiotherapy. *Integr. Cancer Ther.* **6**, 242–250.

Chattha, R., Nagarathna, R., Padmalatha, V. and Nagendra, H.R. (2008) Effect of yoga on cognitive functions in climacteric syndrome: A randomized control study. *B J O G* **115**, 991–1000.

Chattha, R., Raghuram, N., Venkatram, P. and Hongasandra, N.R. (2008) Treating the climacteric symptoms in Indian women with an integrated approach to yoga therapy: A randomized control study. *Menopause* **15**, 862–870.

Chaya, M.S., Ramakrishnan, G., Shastry, S., Kishore, R.P., Nagendra, H., Nagarathna, R., Raj, T., Thomas, T., Vaz, M. and Kurpad, A.V. (2008) Insulin sensitivity and cardiac autonomic function in young male practitioners of yoga. *Natl. Med. J. India* **21**, 217–221.

Datey, K.K., Deshmukh, S., Dalvi, C. and Vinekar, S.L. (1969) "Shavasan": A yogic exercise in the management of hypertension. *Angiology* **20**, 325–333.

Descilo, T., Vedamurtachar, A., Gerbarg, P.L., Nagaraja, D., Gangadhar, B.N., Damodaran, B., Adelson, B., Braslow, L.H., Marcus, S. and Brown, R.P. (2009) Effects of a yoga breath intervention alone and in combination with an exposure therapy for post-traumatic stress disorder and depression in survivors of the 2004 South-East Asia tsunami. *Acta. Psychiatr. Scand.* **121**(4), 289–300.

Desiraju, T. (1983) Neurophsiology and consciousness. An integrated non-dualist evolutionary theory. In: *Frontiers in Physiological Research*. Garlick, D.G., Korner, P., (eds.) Cambridge University Press Cambridge, New York.

Duraiswami, G., Thirthalli, J., Nagendra, H.R. and Gangadhar, B.N. (2007) Yoga therapy as an add-on treatment in the management of patients with schizophrenia — a randomized controlled trial. *Acta. Psychitry. Scand.* **116**, 226–232.

Janakiramaiah, N., Gangadhar, B.N., Naga Venkatesha Murthy, P.J., Harish, M.G., Subbakrishna, D.K. and Vedamurthachar, A. (2000) Antidepressant efficacy of Sudarshan Kriya Yoga (SKY) in melancholia: A randomized comparison with electroconvulsive therapy (ECT) and imipramine. *J. Affect. Disord.* **57**, 255–259.

Khalsa, S.B., Khalsa, G.S., Khalsa, H.K. and Khalsa, M.K. (2008) Evaluation of a residential Kundalini yoga lifestyle pilot program for addiction in India. *J. Ethn. Subst. Abuse.* **7**, 67–79.

Kochupillai, V., Kumar, P., Singh, D., Aggarwal, D., Bhardwaj, N., Bhutani, M. and Das, S.N. (2005) Effect of rhythmic breathing (Sudarshan kriya and Pranayama) on immune functions and tobacco addiction. *Ann. N.Y. Acad. Sci.* **1056**, 242–252.

Krishnamurthy, M. and Telles, S. (2007b) Effects of yoga and an ayurveda preparation on gait, balance and mobility in older persons. *Med. Sci. Monit.* **13**, 19–20.

Krishnamurthy, M.N. and Telles, S. (2007a) Assessing depression following two ancient Indian interventions: Effects of yoga and ayurveda on older adults in a residential home. *J. Gerontol. Nurs.* **33**, 17–23.

Kuvalayananda, S. (1925) X-ray experiments on Uddiyana and Nauli in relation to the position of the colonel contents. *Yoga Mimansa* **1**, 250–254.

Malathi, A. and Damodaran, A. (1999) Stress due to exams in medical students — role of yoga. *Indian J. Physiol. Phrmacol.* **43**, 218–224.

Manchanda, S.C., Narang, R., Reddy, K.S., Sachdeva, U., Prabhakaran, D., Dharmanand, S., Rajani, M. and Bijlani, R. (2000) Retardation of coronary atherosclerosis with yoga lifestyle intervention. *J. Assoc. Physicians India.* **48**, 687–694.

Manjunath, N.K. and Telles, S. (2005) Influence of yoga and ayurveda on self-rated sleep in a geriatric population. *Indian J. Med. Res.* **121**, 683–690.

Manjunath, N.K. and Telles, S. (2006) Pulmonary functions following yoga in a community dwelling geriatric population in India. *J. Indian Psychol.* **24**, 17–25.

Nagarathna, R. and Nagendra, H.R. (1985) Yoga for bronchial asthma: A controlled study. *Br. Med. J.* **291**, 1077–1079.

Ornish, D., Scherwitz, L.W., Billings, J.H., Brown, S.E., Gould, K.L., Merritt, T.A., Sparler, S., Armstrong, W.T., Ports, T.A., Kirkeeide, R.L., Hogeboom, C. and Brand, R.J. (1998) Intensive lifestyle changes for reversal of coronary heart disease. *J. AM. Med. Assoc.* **280**, 2001–2007. Erratum in: *J. AM. Med. Assoc.* (1999) **281**, 1380.

Patel, C. (1975) 12-month follow-up yoga and bio-feedback in the management of hypertension. *Lancet* **11**, 62–64.

Patel, C. and North, W.R. (1975) Randomised controlled trial of yoga and bio-feedback in management of hypertension. *Lancet* **19**, 93–95.

Raghavendra, R.M., Nagarathna, R., Nagendra, H.R., Gopinath, K.S., Srinath, B.S., Ravi, B.D., Patil, S., Ramesh, B.S. and Nalini R. (2007) Effects of an integrated yoga programme on chemotherapy-induced nausea and emesis in breast cancer patients. *Eur. J. Cancer Care* **16**, 462–474.

Rao, R.M., Telles, S., Nagendra, H.R., Nagarathna, R., Gopinath, K., Srinath, S. and Chandrashekhara, C. (2008) Effects of yoga on natural killer cell counts in early breast cancer patients undergoing conventional treatment. *Med. Sci. Monit.* **13**, 3–4.

Rawal, S.B., Singh, M.V., Tyagi, A.K., Selvamurthy, W. and Chaudhuri, B.N. (1994) Effect of yogic exercise on thyroid function in subjects resident at sea level upon exposure to high altitude. *Int. J. Biometeorol.* **38**, 188–193.

Sahay, B.K. (2007) Role of yoga in diabetes. *J. Assoc. Physicians India* **55**, 121–126.

Sahay, B.K. and Sahay, R.K. (2002) Lifestyle modification in management of diabetes mellitus. *J. Indian Med. Assoc.* **100**, 178–180.

Sathyaprabha, T.N., Satishchandra, P., Pradhan, C., Sinha, S., Kaveri, B., Thennarasu, K., Murthy, B.T. and Raju, T.R. (2008) Modulation of cardiac autonomic balance with adjuvant yoga therapy in patients with refractory epilepsy. *Epilepsy Behav.* **12**, 245–252.

Selvamurthy, W., Ray, U.S., Hegde, K.S. and Sharma, R.P. (1988) Physiological responses to cold (10 degrees C) in men after six months' practice of yoga exercises. *Int. J. Biometeorol.* **32**, 188–193.

Sharma, V.K., Das, S., Mondal, S., Goswami, U. and Gandhi, A. (2006) Effect of Sahaj yoga on neuro-cognitive functions in patients suffering from major depression. *Indian J. Physiol. Pharmacol.* **50**, 375–383.

Sharma, V.K., Das, S., Mondal, S., Goswami, U. and Gandhi, A. (2005) Effect of Sahaj yoga on depressive disorders. *Indian J. Physiol. Pharmacol.* **49**, 462–468.

Singh, V. (1987) Kunjal: A nonspecific protactive factor in management of bronchial asthma. *J. Asthma.* **24**, 183–186.

Singh, V., Wisniewski, A., Britton, J. and Tattersfeld, A. (1990) Effect of yoga breathing exercises (pranayama) on airway reactivity in subjects with asthma. *Lancet* **335**, 1381–1383.

Subramanyam, S., Satyanarayana, M. and Rajeshwari K.R. (1986) Alcoholism: Newer methods of management. *Indian J. Physiol. Pharmacol.* **30**, 43–54.

Telles, S. and Desiraju, T. (1993) Autonomic changes in Brahmakumaris Raja yoga meditation. *Int. J. Psychophysiol.* **5**, 147–152.

Telles, S. and Naveen, K.V. (2006) Effect of yoga on somatic indicators of distress in professional computer users. *Med. Sci. Monit.* **12**, 21–22.

Telles, S., Dash, M. and Naveen, K.V. (2008) Effect of yoga on musculoskeletal discomfort and motor functions in professional computer users. *Work* **33**, 1–10.

Telles, S., Gaur, V. and Balkrishna, A. (2009) Effects of a yoga practice session and a yoga theory session on state anxiety. *Percept. Mot. Skills.* **109**(3), 924–930.

Telles, S., Joseph, C., Venkatesh, S. and Desiraju, T. (1993) Alternations of auditory middle latency evoked potentials during yogic consciously regulated breathing and attentive state of mind. *Int. J. Psychophysiol.* **14**, 189–198.

Telles, S., Naveen, K.V. and Balkrishna, A. (2010) Serum leptin, cholesterol and glucose levels in diabetics following a yoga and diet change program. *Med. Sci. Monit.* **16**(3), LE4–5.

Telles, S., Naveen, K.V. and Dash, M. (2007) Yoga reduces symptoms of distress in tsunami survivors in the Andaman Islands. *Evid. Based Complement. Alternat. Med.* **4**, 218–224.

Telles, S., Naveen, K.V., Dash, M., Deginal, R. and Manjunath, N.K. (2006) Effect of yoga on self-rated visual discomfort in computer users. *Head Face Med.* **3**, 46.

Telles, S., Naveen, K.V., Kumar, N. and Balkrishna, A. (2010) The effect of yoga on neuroticism in an Indian population varies with sociodemographic factors. *J. Cult. Divers* (in press).

Telles, S., Naveen, V.K., Balkrishna, A. and Kumar, S. (2010) Short term health impact of a yoga and diet change program on obesity. *Med. Sci. Monit.* **16**(1), CR35–40.

Vedamurthachar, A., Janakiramaiah, N., Hegde, J.M., Shetty, T.K., Subbakrishna, D.K., Sureshbabu, S.V. and Gangadhar, B.N. (2006) Antidepressant efficacy and hormonal effects of Sudarshana Kriya Yoga (SKY) in alcohol dependent individuals. *J. Affect. Disord.* **94**, 249–253.

Visweswaraiah, N.K. and Telles, S. (2004) Randomized trial of yoga as a complementary therapy for pulmonary tuberculosis. *Respirology* **9**, 96–101.

Vyas, R., Raval, K.V. and Dikshit, N. (2008) Effect of Raja yoga meditation on the lipid profile of post-menopausal women. *Indian J. Physiol. Pharmacol.* **52**, 420–424.

Wallace, R.K. (1970) Physiological effects of transcendental meditation. *Science* **167**, 1751–1754.

Wenger, M.A., Bagchi, B.K. and Anand, B.K. (1961) Experiments in India on "voluntary" control of the heart and pulse. *Circulation* **24**, 1319–1325.

Yogendra, J., Yogendra, H.J., Ambardkar, S., Lele, R.D., Shetty, S., Dave, M. and Husein, N. (2004) Beneficial effects of yoga lifestyle on reversibility of ischaemic heart disease: Caring heart project of International Board of Yoga. *J. Assoc. Physicians India* **52**, 283–289.

Yogi, M.M. (1966) *The Science of Being and the Art of Living.* International SRM Publications, London 1966.

Index

Index